Contents

PART TWO
The Grape Cure

By Johanna Brandt
(abridged and reformatted)

The Detox Mono Diet

"Detoxification is the missing link in Western nutrition, and fasting and/or juice cleansing is a pure and safe form (over water fasting) of detoxification. Dr. Vasey's very informative book brings light to this vital process through one of the first approaches to cleansing, Johanna Brandt's Grape Cure. There are so many people and so many health conditions that can benefit from the natural health approach found in *The Detox Mono Diet*."

ELSON M. HAAS, M.D., THE DETOX DOC
(WWW.ELSONHAAS.COM),
AUTHOR OF *The New Detox Diet* AND
Staying Healthy with Nutrition

"Enthusiastic applause for the combined efforts of Dr. Vasey and the late Mrs. Brandt! Give *The Detox Mono Diet* your full attention, and you will have the foundation for success in self-healing."

CARRIE L'ESPERANCE,
AUTHOR OF *The Seasonal Detox Diet*

"Finally, a fully comprehensive and *accurate* dossier on how to rest the body from complicated combinations of foods—and enable a return to vibrant health. *The Detox Mono Diet* is inspiring and scientifically sound."

NATALIA ROSE,
AUTHOR OF *The Raw Food Detox Diet*

ALSO BY CHRISTOPHER VASEY, N.D.

The Acid–Alkaline Diet for Optimum Health
Restore Your Health by Creating pH Balance in Your Diet

The Water Prescription
For Health, Vitality, and Rejuvenation

The Whey Prescription
The Healing Miracle in Milk

The
Detox
Mono
Diet

The Miracle
Grape Cure
and Other
Cleansing Diets

Christopher Vasey, N.D.

Translated by Jon E. Graham

Healing Arts Press
Rochester, Vermont

Healing Arts Press
One Park Street
Rochester, Vermont 05767
www.HealingArtsPress.com

Healing Arts Press is a division of Inner Traditions International

Originally published in French under the title *Les cures de santé: Régénération et détoxication: L'exemple de la cure de raisin* by Éditions Jouvence, S.A., Chemin du Guillon 20, Case 143, CH-1233 Genève-Bernex, Switzerland, www.editions-jouvence.com, info@editions-jouvence.com

First U.S. edition published in 2006 by Healing Arts Press

Note to the reader: This book is intended as an informational guide. The remedies, approaches, and techniques described herein are meant to supplement, and not to be a substitute for, professional medical care or treatment. They should not be used to treat a serious ailment without prior consultation with a qualified health care professional.

LIBRARY OF CONGRESS CATALOGING-IN-PUBLICATION DATA
Vasey, Christopher.
   [Cures de santé. English]
   The detox mono diet : the miracle grape cure and other cleansing diets / Christopher Vasey ; translated by Jon E. Graham.
      p. cm.
   "Originally published in French under the title : Les cures de santé. Genève-Bernex : Éditions Jouvence, S.A."
   Summary: "An introduction to the healing effects of fasting using just one type of food"—Provided by publisher.
   Includes bibliographical references and index.
   ISBN-13: 978-1-59477-126-2 (pbk.)
   ISBN-10: 1-59477-126-X (pbk.)
   1. Diet therapy—Popular works. 2. Detoxification (Health) I. Title.
   RM237.9.V37 2006
   615.8'54—dc22
                                                                    2006016442

Printed and bound in Canada by Transcontinental Printing

10   9   8   7   6   5   4   3   2

Text design by Priscilla Baker
Text layout by Virginia Scott Bowman
This book was typeset in Sabon with Avenir as the display typeface

Foreword

The book that you are about to read is a harbinger. It represents the result of extensive work done by one woman on her own body during the 1920s. This exceptional woman, Johanna Brandt, was then a nurse living in South Africa.

This book reminds us of the long path traveled by those who have gone before us, the difficulties they encountered—and overcame—as well as victories won by those with strong, clear motivation.

A new paradigm, a conceptual context—perhaps a better description would be a "pair of glasses" that inspires us at the threshold of a new millennium to look anew at health, illness, the individual, and his environment—was already at work with Brandt. This steadfast and visionary woman, eager to share what she had experienced, was in the avantgarde of a wave that has swept across the West, a wave that can be described as the "holistic approach," or global approach.

Essentially, from the holistic perspective, health is no longer viewed as the absence of illness nor the opposite of illness. Health is neither a right nor a product to be bought, but is rather a personal and collective itinerary, an individual journey. It is:

> a movement toward self-mastery and control over one's relationship to oneself, to others and to an ever expanding environment, toward clarity, autonomy, and the discovery of an increasingly satisfying personal insight.[1]

From this perspective, people stricken by an illness can be "healthy" nonetheless if they understand their illness and they have mastered the long-term treatments required to maintain balance.

Illness of any kind can also be a growth experience; it can inspire one to reorganize priorities in life and encourage the experience of self-reassessment and openness to a larger spiritual dimension.

Brandt was wise enough to listen to her inner guide, to become a purposeful and autonomous woman confronting the illness that had struck her. She sought to learn all she could about it, she listened, and she personally tested the Grape Cure with notable success. It enabled her to heal herself and, later, inspired her to share what she had learned.

In her book she wrote:

> Nothing has been said in this article about the mental aspect of healing. The subject is too big. It forms the most thrilling story of my life, but I must be now content to state that I became super-conscious. I had unerring "hunches" and cultivated a bowing acquaintance with my subliminal self—whatever that may be.

Almost eighty years ago, Brandt described the importance of each patient taking responsibility for his or her illness, and of remaining open to the inner guide, the healer we all carry within ourselves.

Brandt did not resist sharing her discovery of the grape diet and its effects. Spurred on by a desire to provide help and comfort, she successfully publicized the regimen that had contributed so much to her own healing. Today, almost everyone who boasts knowledge of alternative approaches to health will understand the beneficial properties of the grape as an example of a mono diet cure.

Between 1927 and 2006, an explosion of health-related knowledge attained dimensions never before imagined. Brandt wrote her book using the terminology in vogue at the time. Scientists today seek a better understanding of Brandt's theories to support acceptance of her hypothesis regarding the Grape Cure's singular effectiveness.

This is what Christopher Vasey has accomplished. The first part of the book prepares the way for Brandt's findings by discussing the importance of the physical environment in which illness and toxins exist. It offers particularly useful information about fasting, autolysis, and mono diets in general. Further on, the author discusses the virtues of grapes, of raw food diets, and, most importantly, addresses the indications and contraindications of a grape mono diet.

So many people interested in the Grape Cure as a preventive health measure—or as a healing strategy against a serious illness—will find precise information here to help them successfully follow this cure. They will also find a wealth of scientific data explaining the reasons behind the effectiveness of this cure.

Of course, the human being is part of a whole, a global unit, and the Grape Cure cannot be solely responsible for healing serious illness. In addition to the healing properties provided by grapes, this cure represents an enormous effort of will. It requires a decision, a willingness to take responsibility for one's life and to take charge of reorienting that life in a way that assists the body in its struggle against an invader.

Those who undertake a Grape Cure accept the requirements to change, to remain receptive, and to believe in the results. In other words, they act as "an exceptional patient"—as described by Dr. Bernie Siegel in his book *Love, Medicine, and Miracles*—as "care users" who dare to affirm themselves and follow through to the end of what they expect will make them well. Thus they care for the body and the mind.

The Detox Mono Diet is now available for those who want to learn more about healing themselves.

Several years before his death, the psychologist Carl Rogers wrote:

You know I believe that no one has ever taught anybody anything. I question the effectiveness of teaching. The only thing I know is that he who wants to learn will learn. Any powerful teacher is a facilitator, a person who brings things to the table and shows people how appetizing and wonderful they are, and then tells them to serve themselves.

This is what Brandt and Vasey do for you. So serve yourself and walk to your own rhythm to reach a higher level of well-being.

That is what I sincerely wish for you.

ROSETTE POLETTI, ADJUNCT DIRECTOR
OF THE SWISS RED CROSS COLLEGE OF NURSING

Introduction

The Grape Cure, the lemon cure, the maple syrup cure . . . the apple mono diet, the rice mono diet, the carrot mono diet . . . the separate foods diet, Dr. X's diet, and so on—patients who seek healing by following a health regimen have an embarrassment of riches to choose from. Health cures are numerous and their promoters offer guarantees of exceptional, sometimes miraculous success even for illnesses often considered incurable (such as certain kinds of cancer).

With numerous examples of successful healing combined with advanced theoretical arguments to demonstrate the solid grounds of whatever cure is in question, many people are inspired to follow such cures. However, lively polemics often erupt between the partisans of one cure and those of another. Every cure boasts its adherents and ardent defenders, but also its opponents.

The novice cannot help but be thrown off balance by the conflicting advice he will hear when considering a wide array of cures. How is one to choose from among so many options? And what to make of the fact that, despite their glaring differences, they all arrive at the same result: healing the patient?

The novice will be even more unsettled to learn of cures that were carefully followed and yet a patient's health did not improve but instead grew worse, requiring weeks to recover from the effects of the cure itself.

Faced with situations like these, doubts emerge concerning the effectiveness of cures in general, and a person may reject all health cures. But rejection is unjustified. Unsatisfactory results do not derive from the failure of the cure itself, but rather because the patient erred in the choice of a cure. In other words, the cure in question was not adapted to the needs and characteristics of the patient, and circumstances required a different cure.

Health cures are, in fact, different methods to attain the same goal. Each possesses distinguishing characteristics that make it more effective for certain patients and certain temperaments. But beyond their differences, the healing processes triggered by these cures are the same and function identically.

The purpose of this book is to show this unity so that patients can be fully informed when choosing an appropriate cure. More than that, this information can enable motivated patients to design their own cure and modify it over time to meet new situations and new problems that arise.

To realize the many benefits of health cures, patients must understand exactly what processes are triggered and why these processes encourage healing. Rather than presenting this information in a theoretical and abstract manner, I offer it through the example of one cure, perhaps the best known and most practiced in our time: Johanna Brandt's Grape Cure.

The first part of this book thus discusses the Grape Cure in the context of natural medicine, according to concepts of health and sickness as laid down by Hippocrates in the fourth century BCE and, more recently, by Dr. Paul Carton.* We will then examine various procedures in detail (fasting, mono diets, raw food diets, cleansings, and so forth) that are aspects of the Grape Cure, allowing the reader to grasp where the effectiveness of each cure resides and what curative factors they all share.

The complex and challenging moments of the cure (healing crises and detoxification crises) are also presented with care, so the person using the cure can correctly interpret reactions that are triggered within the body and avoid complications and problems. The first section of the book ends with a practical summary of the important points to consider during a health cure.

The second section consists of Brandt's book *The Grape Cure,* in which she recounts her discovery and describes how to follow this cure. Shining through each line is her enthusiasm for the benefits of a cure so simple yet effective—even for acute illness.

Her original book comprised several articles and texts assembled into one work. To avoid excessive repetition and to regroup the information she provides, the original text has been lightly abridged and reorganized.

In effect, what the reader holds before him is actually two books: the first explains the "why" of health cures; the second, Brandt's book, explains the "how."

---

*Paul Carton (1875–1947) was a French physician who promoted "naturist vegetarianism." His philosophies were shaped by his own experience of being treated for tuberculosis as a young man. Carton's ideas about the importance of purifying diets of natural foods became quite influential through his writings on the subject.

Part One

DETOXIFICATION AND REGENERATION

1

The True Nature of Illnesses and Therapy

Johanna Brandt was born in South Africa in 1876. Her father was a Dutch pastor; her mother was of French descent. During the harsh Boer War, which raged in South Africa during the early 1900s, Johanna became deeply involved in volunteer nursing. Not without danger to herself, she was able to conduct important "resistance" operations such as transmitting messages and providing supplies to the combatants, as well as providing them shelter and even hiding them when necessary.

She, too, married a pastor, with whom she raised seven children while continuing to lead an active life. During the course of World War I, she was diagnosed with a severe stomach cancer. In 1921, her doctors gave her only six weeks to live. Her desire to survive was so strong that even this somber news did not overwhelm her.

She refused all surgery and courageously set out in search of a cure. She had heard high praise for the benefits of fasting; tangible progress was rapidly achieved when she tried it on herself. By experimenting on her own body this way, she discovered the marvelous healing properties of the grape.

She attributed her complete recovery from cancer to the periods of fasting she practiced at the beginning of her regimen and to the Grape Cure she followed later. The extensively researched and progressive food diet she perfected enabled her to live and enjoy excellent health for another forty years. Until her dying day, at the age of eighty-seven, this amazing woman maintained total vitality.

This was how Mira Dunant-Brandt, Johanna Brandt's daughter, recounted her mother's life to us.

The cancerous tumor that afflicted Brandt was diagnosed clinically and radiologically. Based on the diagnosis, every doctor consulted advised surgery as soon as possible. There was no doubt the tumor was present. The fact that doctors gave her only six more weeks to live testifies to the seriousness of her condition.

And yet Brandt recovered without an operation, using her own means, and lived for another forty years. The simple and natural means she discovered to address her illness gave birth to the Grape Cure, a cure that is now known throughout the world. Thousands and thousands of patients since then have followed her prescription and been cured.

Considering its simplicity and the amazing results it procures, one cannot help but wonder: Why is the Grape Cure so effective? What makes it effective not only against cancer but against numerous other illnesses as well? Routinely, a remedy will work well against a specific disease but not against others. With the grape, the opposite is true; the possibilities for effective action are varied and extensive. This raises the question: Are we dealing with a remedy that has numerous effects, or do these illnesses have a common nature?

Just what is this mysterious and powerful property of the

grape? And why is it the grape that works this way and not some other fruit or vegetable—or, more pointedly, a medicinal herb? Brandt speaks of a mysterious healing substance that the grape must contain—something yet undiscovered in her day that remains unknown even now. But here again, if the identity of this substance were to be discovered, a mystery would remain, because at present we know of no product with such a wide and diverse range of action: destruction of cancerous cells, reduction of painful inflammation in the joints, cure of tuberculosis, prevention of tooth and hair loss, treatment of anemia, regeneration of necrotic or dying tissue, and so forth.

The Grape Cure is disturbing by the number of questions it raises. It calls into question so many medical concepts regarded as certain and definitive. Frankly, why does the grape succeed where more sophisticated remedies fail? To be sure, we can agree that with modern medications, while they provide relief to cancer and rheumatism sufferers, for example, they rarely cure them!

Any attempt to deny the reality of the Grape Cure must ignore the factual evidence. For example, tens of thousands of patients have been cured of a host of illnesses with its help. Tens of thousands more could be cured by applying it sensibly. The results are observable and reproducible and should, therefore, be scientifically acceptable.

Rather than deny the cure's effectiveness, it would be better to find out why it is effective. This would open new vistas, new ways to understand how the body functions and the role played by illness in this function. Therapeutic science—in other words, possibilities for the art of healing—would be enriched with new methods for positive treatment of the sick.

On many occasions, Brandt spoke of toxic substances that make us ill, whereas many people believe that germs make us sick. So, which is it? What is the actual cause of illness, germs or the poisons about which Brandt speaks?

ARE GERMS THE CAUSE OF ILLNESS?

First we must note that many illnesses are known to have no microbial cause—germs are not involved in these illnesses either directly or remotely. Furthermore, any attempt at therapeutic disinfecting (such as the use of antibiotics) will have no effect on the course of these illnesses.

Examples of such diseases are: diabetes, asthma, cancer, heart attack, anemia, rickets, migraine, allergies, depression, digestive disorders, circulatory disorders, hormonal disorders, nervous disorders, and the majority of rheumatisms.

Clearly, many illnesses do not involve germs and many serious illnesses are among their number.

Of course, germ activity is evident at times. Their presence is visible in bronchitis, pneumonia, colds, flu, cystitis, gonorrhea, hepatitis, AIDS, nephritis, and so forth.

Because observation repeatedly confirmed the presence of germs in so-called infectious diseases, an apparently logical conclusion was that germs cause these illnesses. In other words, it was enough for germs simply to enter the body for illness to establish itself.

This may come as a surprise to some, but this deduction contains an error. Of course germs can trigger illness; they *can* do it, but it is not inevitable that they *will* do it. Furthermore, even those germs that do cause illness will not do so in every case. History has shown that during epidemics of the flu and other diseases, not everyone who comes into contact with the disease will contract it. If the mere presence of the germ were enough to trigger illness every time, then epidemics of typhus, cholera, plague, yellow fever, Spanish flu, measles, polio, and so on would have long since wiped the human race off the face of the globe. In actuality, during any epidemic, only a portion of the population is stricken. Others resist the infection; their physical defenses prevent the germs from surviving inside their bodies, where the microbes would otherwise develop and demonstrate their destructive capabilities.

So it appears that germs are not the only factors to be considered. The body's state of receptivity and resistance must also be taken into account. The relative strength of these two factors—the strength of the germs and that of the body's power to resist them—determines whether or not an illness can take hold. The weaker the body's defenses, the easier it will be for germs to gain a foothold and multiply, thus causing illness. In contrast, the more resistant the body's internal cellular environment is, the harder for germs to survive and take action in an environment they find unfavorable.

The body's internal cellular characteristics—whether positive or negative—are not only the determining factors in whether or not a disease will take hold; depending on the germ involved, this internal environment may also determine the form an illness will take. In other words, the nature of an illness that appears may be more dependent on the body's weakness than on the attacking microbe. A great many microbes are not specific; for example, a streptococcus can, depending on the internal cellular environment it has penetrated, cause an angina, internal inflammation, blood poisoning, scarlet fever, or a skin infection. A pneumococcus can cause a herpes vesicle as well as pneumonia or meningitis, all depending on the state of the cellular environment it has entered.

The predominance of intercellular environment over germ is demonstrated also by the fact that the same illness can be caused by different microbes. Bronchitis, angina, and flu can all be caused by cocci as well as by bacilli and viruses.

Germs

Germs are not the primary cause of illness. On the one hand, numerous nonmicrobial diseases are known to exist, and on the other hand, the possibility that germs will cause an infectious illness is subordinate to the strength or weakness of the body's defense system.

These examples demonstrate clearly the importance of the receiver (the body) over the received (the germ).

Although natural medicine considers the internal cellular environment to be the primary factor in illness, this does not ignore the harm done by germs. Germs, viruses, and parasites are real and represent potential dangers to the human body, though considering them the primary cause of disease is a mistake.

The preeminent role of the internal cellular environment over the germ was also recognized by Louis Pasteur, the French researcher to whom we credit the discovery of germs and their action, as well as the realization of the first vaccines. It is widely reported that on his deathbed, Louis Pasteur acknowledged the position of his detractors—those who contested his view that germs alone were responsible for infectious disease and who completed his theory regarding the physical environment's receptivity or resistance to germs. The phrase attributed to Pasteur on his deathbed has since become famous: "The germ is nothing, the internal environment is everything."

WHAT IS THE INTERNAL CELLULAR ENVIRONMENT?

Why does the internal cellular environment play such a deciding role in health? What is it exactly?

The internal cellular environment consists of all the fluids that irrigate the body and in which the cells are immersed. This includes blood circulating in veins and arteries as well as in capillaries, which are the hair-thin vessels that permeate tissue; *lymph,* the "white blood" circulating in lymphatic vessels and nodes; and the *extracellular* and *intracellular fluids* that surround and fill the cells.

Cells cannot move about on their own either in search of nourishment or to expel waste. To achieve these tasks, they depend on these bodily fluids, which function as transporters.

Nutritive substances like vitamins and minerals, but also necessary oxygen, are first transported by blood and lymph, then by cellular fluids to their final destination: the cells. Cellular wastes follow the same path in reverse to exit the body.

In this way, cells draw what they need from bodily fluids, but they also must release their wastes into the fluids.

So bodily fluids are simultaneously a nourishing environment and a system for eliminating toxins. The composition of these fluids constantly changes as a function of the normal or abnormal presence of nutrients and toxins. An overly high concentration of toxins—or, conversely, a deficiency of nutrients—will change internal cellular characteristics and alter the cells' ability to function.

The Internal Cellular Environment

This environment consists of all bodily fluids (blood, lymph, cellular fluids) that irrigate the body and also bathe the cells. The ideal composition of the internal cellular environment can be changed by a surcharge of toxins or a deficiency of nutrients, or even both happening together.

The composition of physical fluids—in other words, the characteristics of the internal cellular environment—thus sets the stage for the body to stay healthy or fall ill. *Everything depends on the internal cellular environment.* Whatever illnesses a person may suffer, the effects are not confined to localized symptoms, but are connected to a deep overall imbalance caused by deficiencies in the internal cellular environment. It could not be otherwise. This environment provides the condition for symptoms to emerge, and not the other way around.

As we have seen, the role of germs in the genesis of these deficiencies is secondary. So what, then, is the role played by toxins in the appearance of diseases?

ILLNESSES AND TOXINS

When Brandt speaks of the causes of disease, she does not refer to germs but always to poisons, toxic substances, and wastes. Do the facts confirm her point of view? As we can see for ourselves, this is precisely the case. Observation of illness reveals, in all diseases, the presence of an internal cellular environment that is to some degree overburdened with toxins.

Phlegm encumbers the pulmonary alveoli in asthma, the bronchial tubes in bronchitis, the throat when one coughs, the sinus in sinusitis, and the nose during a cold. When people suffering from respiratory ailments cough, expectorate, and blow their noses, they are trying to rid themselves of wastes stagnating in their respiratory tracts.

Grit and crystalline precipitates inflame, block, and deform the joints of arthritis and rheumatism sufferers.

Colloidal wastes (aggregates made up of waste substances) are eliminated by the sebaceous glands in the form of acne, boils, and sweat-induced eczema. Crystalline or acidic wastes are expelled by the sweat glands in the form of dry eczema, chapped skin, and pruritus (itching).

Excess food substances present in the stomach and intestines cause regurgitation, indigestion, nausea, vomiting, or diarrhea. When these substances act as irritants, or they ferment or putrefy, they cause inflammation of digestive mucous membranes (gastritis, enteritis, colitis), and the manufacture of gas (flatulence, bloating).

Cholesterol and excess fatty acids are the culprits in cardiovascular diseases, to which 37 percent of all U.S. deaths in 2003 were attributed.[1] These substances thicken the blood and form deposits on vessel walls (atherosclerosis), deform vessel walls (varicose veins), inflame them (phlebitis, arteritis), and obstruct them (infarction, stroke, pulmonary embolism).

In allergies, the guilty substances are allergens (substances that induce allergic reactions); in kidney disease, they are protein wastes; in obesity, fats; in diabetes, sugar; in gout, uric acid; in osteoporosis, acids; and in cancer—the disease Brandt contracted that led to her discovery of the Grape Cure—carcinogens, substances implicated in promoting the development of cancer.

Toxins are present in the mildest and in the most serious illnesses. They impact health both by their number (the quantitative aspect) and by their properties (the qualitative aspect).

Quantitatively, when a significant mass of waste stagnates in extracellular fluid, the body's cells literally bathe in a swamp that paralyzes all exchanges. Oxygen and nutritive substances make their way to the cells with great difficulty. It is equally difficult for cellular wastes to move out of the area, and their presence further disturbs the internal cellular environment. The organs containing these cells become congested with wastes and their proper function is compromised. When organs then fail to function, disrupting the body's well-being, we call it sickness. When the liver is congested, we speak of hepatic disorders; pulmonary catarrh (inflammation) indicates an overburdened respiratory tract; kidney stones and gallstones occur when the urinary system is stricken.

On the other hand, some wastes are present only in small quantities, but they have a disproportionately harmful toxic effect. They irritate and inflame tissues (as in rheumatoid arthritis, for example), or they cause lesions and hardening of tissues (as when nervous disorders and motor problems are caused by nerve lesions or multiple sclerosis). Such toxins can also cause alteration of normal cell function, causing cells to behave in ways harmful to the rest of the body (for example, cancerous cells that infiltrate neighboring organs).

> **Toxins**
> Toxins are harmful to health because they congest the organs and poison cells. By accumulating, they create a favorable environment for the development of germs.

Germ activity can increase the harmful effects of toxicity. However, germs can develop only in a degraded internal cellular environment where they combine with wastes that are already manifesting morbid effects. The noxious effect of germs is, moreover, very close to that of toxins, insofar as the emergence of illness is due in large part to poisoning caused by their wastes and the residues they secrete.

Autointoxication (self-poisoning) and congestion of blood and organs thus appear to be the profound nature of illness. This is not a new concept. Although the idea has fallen into disuse, it dates back to remote antiquity and has been a part of the medical tradition of all eras.

THE PROFOUND NATURE OF ILLNESS

According to our ancestors—and this remains valid today—the profound nature of most illness is characterized by the presence of harmful substances in the body. These substances have been identified by a wide variety of names over the years. At present, they are known as toxins. They include cholesterol, uric acid, and crystalline or colloidal wastes. To this list of undesirable substances, we now add food additives (food coloring, preservatives), garden products (herbicides, fungicides, insecticides), medical substances that are administered to livestock (hormones, antibiotics, vaccines), medications we take ourselves (sedatives, sleeping pills, antibiotics), as well as numerous poisons stemming from pollution of the air, earth, and water.

The great doctors of every era have stressed the fundamental role played by poisons. Hippocrates, the father of medicine, wrote: "The nature of all illness is the same. . . . When the contaminated humor is abundant, it will take hold and cast down into sickness all that is healthy. The entire body is attacked and disorganized."[2]

The great English doctor of the seventeenth century Thomas Sydenham (1624–1689) provided a magnificent summary of illness when he said: "A disease, however much its cause may be adverse to the human body, is nothing more than an effort of Nature, who strives with might and main to restore the health of the patient by the elimination of the morbific [disease-causing] humor."[3]

Closer to the present, Dr. Paul Carton—the Hippocrates of the twentieth century—confirmed that "disease in reality is only the translation of an inner effort to neutralize and clean out toxins, which the body performs for preservation and regeneration."[4]

Rudolf Steiner, the founder of a new and unique medicine—anthroposophical medicine—observed that internal ailments stem from the fact that "undesirable substances are dissolving into our fluid being."

Whatever the terminology employed or the era when used, the cause of disease has always been recognized as a buildup of substances that clog bodily tissues. This clogging disrupts the system, and illness is a state of poor organ function created by the presence of these undesirable substances. Disease is not, as is too often perceived, a pre-existing external entity that makes the body sick by entering it. *It is imperative that we do not think of disease as an enemy inside of us and our bodies as battlefields.* Deficiencies in our internal environment, and the poor state of our own bodies, are the fundamental problems we need to work on. From this perspective, *therapy is less like combat waged against an enemy than help brought to a friend in trouble.*

In every disease, we must deal with problems caused by clogged tissues and the body's attempt to neutralize and expel undesirable substances. A double component exists: symptoms brought on by the presence of wastes and symptoms stemming from the body's defense system reacting to the internal environment. In fact, when confronted by an overburdened internal cellular environment—a threat to its existence—the body will not remain a passive spectator. It reacts and seeks to rid itself of undesirable substances. To do this, the body intensifies the action of filtering organs—emunctory or excretory organs—which include the liver, intestines, skin, and respiratory tract.

For example, the obvious symptoms of bronchitis are due as much to the presence of colloidal wastes that congest the bronchial tubes as they are to the respiratory tract's attempt to protect against these wastes (hypersecretion of mucus by the mucous membranes) and carry them out of the body (expectoration, coughing, asthma crises, inflammation). Rheumatism is a response to aggressive acid wastes that irritate joints and create lesions and pain. But a joint defends itself, which results in heat and congestion in the affected region.

Disease

The profound nature of disease centers on the general deficiencies of the internal cellular environment of the body. Disease symptoms are merely secondary manifestations—superficial and localized—of this deep problem.

If the state of the internal cellular environment is truly responsible for disease, the problem cannot help but be as general as this environment. This global approach to illness contrasts to the current fragmented model that treats illness as a localized disorder, confined to a specific region of the body. From such a perspective, a person suffering from painful joints has sick joints only; the rest of the body is not ill. It follows that a cancer sufferer is stricken only at the site of the cancerous tissue; an eczema sufferer at the level of the skin; the constipated individual has a problem with intestines alone; and so forth.

It is surprising that anyone would suggest diseases limit themselves to isolated regions of the body, considering the interdependence of organs and the fact that body fluids (blood, lymph, serum) are in constant circulation, which means nutritive substances and poisons alike are distributed throughout the internal cellular environment. To believe that wastes accumulate only in the diseased region of the body hardly conforms to physiology. People with an acne outbreak localized at their upper back do not carry wastes only in this area of tissue; waste collects throughout their internal cellular environment. Excessive wastes spill over and become visible in the afflicted area as the body attempts to rid itself of toxins. A cancer sufferer does not carry toxins only in the neighborhood of a tumor, but in every cell of the body, as evidenced by the fact that, along with symptoms caused by the presence of a tumor, the individual will suffer from additional disorders (digestive, nervous, circulatory, eliminatory, and so on).

Disease—and not its symptoms—is therefore general: it is the buildup of congestion in the body's internal cellular environment. There is no such thing as a localized illness; diseases are always a sign of generalized problems. Given these conditions, what therapy should be applied?

THE FOUNDATIONS OF THERAPY

We are accustomed to using medications that kill germs and cause symptoms to abate. Should we now seek a whole range of medications to destroy each kind of toxin?

Not at all! It is not possible to dispel toxins from the body by destroying them. Destroying toxins means breaking them into smaller pieces; it does not mean they have been reduced to nothing. The internal cellular environment will remain congested with toxic residues, and their presence will remain unaddressed.

The tissues must rid themselves of these toxins stagnating in fluids by expelling them from the body.

The body is equipped with specialized organs designed to extract such wastes from blood and lymph and carry them outside. These are the excretory organs mentioned earlier.

The basic therapy aims at correcting the cellular environment by eliminating excess substances through the excretory organs. "All diseases are resolved either by the mouth, the bowels, the bladder, or some other such organ. Sweat is a common form of resolution in all these cases," writes Hippocrates.[5] In essence, if disease is truly caused by poisons, only detoxification can successfully deal with it.

Draining

Draining is the means by which this cleansing is achieved.

Draining consists of stimulating the body's excretory organs to filter and eliminate toxins. The means—or drainers—that effect this stimulation are varied. They may include the use of medicinal plants, drinking juices or eating foods that have detoxifying properties, adhering to a diet, stimulating reflex zones, applying massage, cleansing the intestines, and using hydrotherapy (specific instructions for attending to these issues can be found in chapters 6 and 7).

The liver, intestines, kidneys, skin, and respiratory tract are the essential pathways through which draining is effected. In draining cures, therapeutic efforts are directed at these organ systems to restore normal elimination or, better, to increase elimination for a period to make up for lost time.

First, the individual excretory organ, when stimulated by one or more drainers, will cleanse itself of wastes that lie stagnant in its tissues and clog its "filter." Once it has been cleansed, the excretory organ will regain its ability to filter blood properly. The blood, in turn, irrigates deep tissues and rids them of accumulated toxins, transporting wastes to the excretory organs.

Draining is thus characterized by increased waste elimination by excretory organs. *This increased elimination will be apparent to the person taking the cure:* material expelled by the intestines will be more abundant or evacuation will occur more regularly. Urine charged with waste will take on a darker color and will increase markedly in volume. The skin will sweat more copiously, and the respiratory tract will free itself of colloidal waste that encumbers it through increased coughing and inflammation.

The level of toxins trapped in tissues will fall with increased elimination. This will cleanse the internal cellular environment and the body's overall health will improve, while symptoms of illness will diminish and gradually disappear. The opportunity for healing obviously depends on how much the body has been damaged by wastes, as well as on the various organs' ability to regenerate. But the principle of detoxification remains valid; the fact that specific local treatments can be added to the basic therapy does not challenge the premise.

If draining toxins was not the logical response to the true nature of illness, how could we explain that for the same patient, a single therapy—the general draining of toxins—can dispel all health problems, despite the vast differences that might characterize the disorders?

A multitude of patients, after running from one specialist to the next to treat various disorders, eventually found themselves cured of *all* conditions by a single causal treatment.

Importance of Maintaining Open Excretory Organs

The excretory organs serve as the obligatory exit doors for toxins. The following figures illustrate the importance of these organs and emphasize the consequences that may result when any of them slow down or lose function.

The kidneys should eliminate 25–30 grams of urea over a twenty-four-hour period. If they eliminate only 20 grams, this represents retention of at least 5 grams per day, or 150 grams ($^1/_3$ pound) per month! These 150 grams of urea will clog the tissues and overburden the internal cellular environment. The same is true for salt. If the kidneys eliminate 12 grams of salt (NaCl) in twenty-four hours, instead of the entire 15 or more grams that are typically absorbed from food, this means 3 grams each day are retained—90 grams per month!

To be sure, these elimination figures are not precise, as wastes can be expelled through more than one exit. Nevertheless, waste substances do accumulate in tissues, as can be seen during dialysis.

During one twenty-four-hour period of blood dialysis—in which all blood is extracted from the body and run through a filter that removes urea before the blood is reintroduced through a vein—one can collect as much as 300–400 grams of urea, whereas the presence of merely a few grams (2 grams per liter of blood) is considered fatal. These 300–400 grams of urea are obviously not stored in the bloodstream; but because they cannot be eliminated by the excretory organs, they are pushed deeper into tissues, where they contribute to congestion of the internal cellular environment.

Recognizing Good Excretory Function

The criteria for good excretory function are as follows: the intestines should empty once a day; the stools should be well formed but not hard and they should not have a nauseating smell. The speed at which food travels through the intestines is also important. Food should leave the body within twenty-four to thirty-six hours after it is eaten. Hard, dry stools that are difficult to expel, are accompanied by a foul odor, and are evacuated every two to three days or more, are a sign of self-poisoning in the intestines, characterized by poor elimination.

Kidneys eliminate approximately 1.3 to 1.5 liters of urine each day. Urine should contain certain wastes that can be detected only through analysis but which give it a typical color and odor. Consequently, a kidney insufficiency is indicated by urine that is too clear, has no color or odor, or is too infrequent (meaning only two or three urinations a day). Urine that is highly charged with wastes testifies to strong elimination capacity, but also reveals a high level of contamination.

The respiratory tract (lungs, bronchi, nasopharynx, sinuses) is a path of elimination for gaseous wastes (CO_2). None of it should be obstructed by solid or fluid wastes (phlegm, mucus, colloidal wastes). If there is congestion, it is a sign that the body as a whole has accumulated too many toxins and is trying to expel some of them through the respiratory tract. Except for a few waste products present when a person rises in the morning, the nose should always be clear and free of congestion.

Therapy

The purpose of therapy is to correct the internal cellular environment and not merely to rid the body of symptoms. Cleansing this environment is achieved through draining and removal of deeply embedded toxins.

With high-volume waste accumulation, draining may not be sufficient and other treatments may be called for. In fact, wastes that are forced deep into tissues will eventually become encrusted and as the buildup increases, they form agglomerations with other wastes, making them difficult to dislodge. Opening the excretory organs and cleansing the blood is not enough to reach them. To clear these accumulations, a therapeutic process must attack the deep-lying toxins where they are concentrated, dislodging and breaking them down into particles that can be picked up by the bloodstream and carried to the excretory organs.

This result cannot be achieved through the use of medications, but the body itself can accomplish it with fasts and highly restrictive diets. In fact, depriving the body of its regular intake of nutritive substances forces it to draw from its own reserves, attack wastes, and break down deposits to obtain those substances it is missing. This breaking down and dislodging of wastes occurs thanks to the action of enzymes, which will be discussed in the next chapter.

A combination of dislodging and draining promotes restoration of the internal cellular environment at the most basic level, and by changing the vital environment of the organs produces healing.

THE HEALING PROCESS AND THE GRAPE CURE

The status one must achieve either to maintain good health or to restore it is the same: one must attain a clean internal cellular environment. To enjoy such a status, one must fight against the buildup of undesirable substances (toxins). Logically, to realize this goal one must:

- Keep the excretory organs "wide open" so that toxins cannot accumulate.
- Periodically increase the filtration and excretion processes of the excretory organs to compensate for potential "delays" in elimination.
- Burn away the encrusted wastes accumulated in the depths of various tissues so they can be carried back toward the surface to the blood and excretory organs for elimination.
- Stimulate the metabolism (conversion of foods to usable substances and energy) in general so that the production of wastes is as limited as possible.
- Maintain the purity of the internal cellular environment by adopting a nontoxic diet that shuts off the source of excess substances.

How does one accomplish these aims? Though clearing the body of toxins has been known to promote incredible healings, by itself the therapy cannot maintain a patient's health. The patient must avoid reintroducing poisons, hence the need to adopt new habits and lifestyles, in particular a hypotoxic diet.

The Grape Cure perfected by Brandt has been so effective and has allowed so many healings because it addresses each of the criteria listed on the previous page.

- Enemas, rubbing, physical exercises, and breathing exercises keep the excretory organs open.
- Eliminations are increased by the depurative (purifying) properties of the grape.
- Fasting breaks down the deep-lying wastes and the diseased cells.
- The unmixed, raw food diet adopted at the end of the cure stimulates the metabolism.
- The final diet is hypotoxic, which interrupts the intake of toxins.

Because the different procedures (fasting, mono diet, raw food diet, avoiding mixing too many foods) and their value are only mentioned but not explained by Brandt, the following chapters will examine these procedures separately, explain how they work, and discuss the healing processes they trigger. This will make it possible to use them advisedly, not only in the Grape Cure, but in whatever other cure one may choose to take.

2
Fasting

To heal herself from cancer, Brandt fasted on numerous occasions. Her fasts lasted from several days to several weeks. She even states bluntly that she sometimes continued them beyond reasonable limits in an attempt to be rid of her tumor.

So what is a fast and how does it work?

A fast is any period during which no food is consumed, only water. During this time, there is no nutritional intake, as water is drunk solely to prevent dehydration. The value of the fast and the effects it produces are due to the complete absence of food intake, which forces the body to function as a closed economy with no external assistance.

The first problem the body must surmount is obviously that of supplying itself with nutritive substances like amino acids, minerals, carbohydrates, and vitamins. These substances are essential for cell survival, organ function, and the repair of cellular wear and tear. But as the body will receive none of these substances from outside during the fast, it will have to find them elsewhere. The sole option is to draw them from within itself.

How does the body achieve this?

AUTOLYSIS

During a fast the body will draw what it needs—nutrients it does not receive from outside—from its own tissues through a process known as autolysis. This is a kind of digestive process—the word literally means digestion (lysis) of one's self (auto). It takes place within the cells, by virtue of enzymes contained in those cells.

Enzymes can be likened to "tiny workers" performing the biochemical transformations the body requires. They are active not only during fasts but at all other times as well. Their work consists of assembling complex substances out of simple substances or dividing complex substances into their component parts. For example, enzymes assemble isolated molecules of glucose to make long chains consisting of more than 10,000 elements: the resulting glycogen is stored in the liver until it's needed for energy. Enzymes also put together amino acids to form proteins, as well as assembling fatty acids and glycerin to make fats. Conversely, their jobs include dividing proteins into amino acids, glycogen into glucose, and so forth. A vast number of different enzymes are at work, each specialized to perform a discrete function.

Enzymes' transformational capacities are apparent in healthy tissue as well as in diseased tissue. They are equally good at breaking down fats stored in healthy reserves as they are at reducing pathological fat accumulations in obese tissue. They will break down muscle proteins as expertly as they deconstruct proteins in cancerous cells, and separate the minerals from bone tissue as well as those contained in a cystic growth.

Autolysis is a natural and common phenomenon. When a splinter is spontaneously pushed out of the body, the tissues that separate it from the surface are gradually digested through autolysis, thus creating a path for the splinter to exit. When the uterus resumes its normal size after a woman gives birth, and when the mammary glands return to their customary size after nursing, these changes occur thanks to the autolytic activity of enzymes.

During a fast, the body digests its own tissue to supply itself with nutrition. The process of autolysis allows the body to survive during a period of privation. However, one can legitimately ask if this process would not be dangerous for the body. In fact, by attacking tissues at random during a fast, would this process risk creating lesions in vital organs such as the heart and the brain, and therefore prompt the faster's death?

Furthermore, with the exceptions of fats and sugars, which are stored specifically for periods when food is scarce, nutritive substances (proteins, minerals, vitamins) are not set aside in special reserves, but are integrated directly into the functioning tissues: into the skeleton, the skin, and the various other organs. Given these circumstances, isn't there cause to fear that by forcing the body to draw nutrients from these tissues, it would deprive them of their constituent elements and thereby make them ill?

Autolysis

Autolysis is a digestive process (lysis) that the body performs on its own (auto) tissues, thanks to enzymatic activity.

THE WISDOM OF
THE BODY AND AUTOLYSIS

Nothing takes place in the body by chance or without reason. To the contrary, everything is directed, triggered, harmonized, and orchestrated in a controlled and intelligent manner. Autolysis is no exception. It does not attack tissues indiscriminately, ravaging everything in its path. People who have practiced fasts, and those who have monitored fasters, have ascertained that the least important tissues are digested before those of greater importance to the body. This fact has been confirmed by studies and research among physiologists.[1]

Over the course of a fast, essential tissues receive necessary nutritive substances thanks to the autolysis of less essential tissues. In other words, the latter are sacrificed for the benefit of the former. For example, proteins and minerals taken from muscles in the arm will be used to nourish the brain. Among these less essential tissues, we not only include muscles, hair, nails, and so forth, contrasted with more critical tissues of the brain, the heart, and the nervous system. We also count among the less essential tissues such things as tumors, goiters, abscesses, growths, pathologically fatty deposits, cellulite, and the like.

To complete the picture, we must also mention nonessential substances like toxins that saturate tissues and congest organs (gluelike substances in bronchial tubes, crystals blocking joints) and toxins circulating in blood and lymph.

Keep in mind that healthy organic tissue, unhealthy tissue, and toxins alike are all built out of nutritive substances brought into the body by food (proteins, minerals). The constituent elements of these can therefore be reutilized through autolysis.

For instance, myomas (tumors of muscular tissue) can provide amino acids; lipomas (tumors of adipose, or fatty, tissue) supply fatty acids; osteomas (tumors of bone tissue) can furnish minerals, and so on. Moreover, cholesterol will supply fatty acids, uric acid provides nitrogenous substances, and the list goes on.

Once a fast has begun, the order in which tissues will be used is as follows: First come the normal "reserves"—glycogen stored in the liver and cells, as well as fat reserves. Once these are exhausted, autolysis will attack tissues that are less important for the body's survival—or when diseased tissue is involved, those that are the most harmful to health. The result is a breakdown of toxins saturating the body's internal cellular environment, as well as destruction of diseased tissue: cysts, tumors, and so on. Autolysis will then proceed to use healthy tissue, starting again with the least essential, such as the muscles. If a fast is continued for too long—during a famine, perhaps—rather than for therapeutic purposes, more and more essential tissue will be autolyzed and eventually death will result from starvation.

Figures that physiologists provide regarding the relative weight loss for each organ in the event of death by starvation—in other words, when fasting is carried to the extreme—reveal the intelligence that governs autolysis of tissues. The losses are listed here in declining order.

Fatty tissue, the body's natural reserves, is depleted the most by this process: 97 percent of the body's fat is broken down by autolysis. Next is the spleen, which loses 67 percent of its initial weight, followed by the liver, which loses 54 percent. These two organs that are so vitally important to the body figure high on the scale because while their loss is large quantitatively, it is of less importance qualitatively.

In fact, water is the primary element eliminated here, in addition to fats and glycogens from the liver. Despite such substantial losses, these organs can continue to function properly.

Next on the list are muscles, which lose 31 percent of their weight; blood, 27 percent (but the tissues it irrigates have also reduced in size); kidneys, 26 percent; skin, 21 percent; lungs, 18 percent; intestines, 18 percent; pancreas, 17 percent; and bones, percent. The organs least affected by autolysis are the brain, spinal cord, and heart, of which only 3 percent of their combined total weight is broken down.

Observing how "nonessential" organs can be autolyzed to supply nutrients to essential organs is impressive in itself. Figures concerning the self-digestion of unhealthy tissue (tumors, cysts) are even more impressive, as these tissues can be autolyzed up to 100 percent.

In other words, pathological tissue can be entirely broken down and destroyed during a fast. Its constituent elements are separated, those that can be reutilized are transported to the organs that need them, and the rest are eliminated. *Thus, a tumor can be entirely purged.*

This is the healing value of a fast. This does not mean that when symptoms of disease disappear (a cancerous tumor, for instance) that a complete cure has been effected. A cure will be realized only when the internal cellular environment that hosted the disease has been corrected and cleansed.

And during a fast—contrasted with many other therapeutic approaches—the internal cellular environment is cleansed. In fact, autolysis of toxins saturating the internal environment takes place in tandem with the autolysis of unhealthy tissue. Thus, for the duration of a fast, not only is the diseased element removed, but the environment that enabled its existence is also cleared. The process described here using the tumor as illustration also applies to other health disorders, including conditions like outbreaks of acne, osteoarthritis, and the flu.

The fact that the body uses waste and diseased tissue before autolyzing healthy tissue makes logical sense. The body, by virtue of its immune system, can distinguish between an integral part of itself and an external element. It can rapidly pinpoint everything that is not "self" or that represents a threat to its physical integrity: for example, intruders (germs, viruses, bacteria, parasites) and poisons and cells that do not conform to the architecture and overall organization of the body (cancerous tissue). Once the body has detected elements that are foreign and harmful, it can organize its immune system to destroy or neutralize "the enemy" selectively.

Breaking down unhealthy tissue is also easier than accessing healthy tissue. The diseased elements are not as well integrated into the overall organic economy of the system and are thus weaker and more easily destroyed.

The point of a therapeutic fast, in the end, is not to push autolysis to create lesions that threaten death. The goal is to trigger the process and maintain it only as long as needed to affect physical cleansing, and always to interrupt autolysis before it damages healthy tissue. The moment when a fast must end is easier to determine than one might suppose: that moment is preceded by the return of *true hunger*. This sensation is a physical hunger that should not be confused with false mental hungers that arise during the fast and are actually a *desire* to eat more than a *need* to eat.

The Intelligence of Autolysis

Autolysis of tissues is achieved intelligently. Essential tissues are not attacked but rather nourished, thanks to the autolysis of tissues that are less essential—or not at all necessary—and to the reuse of toxins they contain, toxins that gradually disappear in this manner over the course of the fast.

TISSUE REGENERATION

Working in tandem with autolysis is a phenomenon known as *tissue regeneration,* also a natural process. Consider the tadpole: common belief holds that tadpoles lose their tails before making the transition to frogs with feet. In reality, they have not lost their tails; they have absorbed them through autolysis. The substances thereby released were used to build feet.

In the human body, too, autolyzed substances are placed at the body's disposal to build new tissue, not merely to repair existing tissue. Because of this, even body growth can continue uninterrupted during a period of fasting. Common observation during the course of a fast reveals that—against all expectations—old wounds scab, badly welded fractures reconsolidate, fresh wounds or ulcers close, and lesions are healed.

Two factors are responsible for this phenomenon of tissue regeneration. On the one hand, autolysis releases substances the body needs to build other tissues. But that factor alone cannot explain the fact of regeneration. After all, during periods of regular food intake, those necessary substances are provided by a normal diet. Something else must be at work here.

The answer is that during a fast, the body gradually rids itself of accumulated wastes, clearing fluids needed for transport, thereby facilitating delivery of nutritive substances to the cells, where they can be put to use. Before a fast, wounds and lesions are immersed in an internal cellular environment saturated with wastes—a kind of swamp obstructing pathways to the cells. Over the course of the fast, toxins are eliminated and the way made clear; minerals and vitamins can once again reach damaged regions to regenerate them.

This regeneration phenomenon also occurs in the blood. Anemic individuals who undertake a fast may see their iron rates climb back to normal. The explanation for this is the same as for other tissue regeneration. Iron is present in the body but is blocked from entering the bloodstream by a congested cellular environment. To be sure, this cure only applies to anemia caused by a deficiency of utilization; it does not apply to anemia caused by intake deficiencies.

Physical Regeneration

During a fast, the body's tissues regenerate and cleanse themselves, but they also repair themselves with the substances that autolysis has provided them.

ELIMINATORY UPDATING

Because all food intake is absent during a fast, the work of the digestive system is eliminated, resulting in considerable energy savings. Digestion, in fact, requires a significant amount of labor from the body. The work of digestion is all the more critical because if the body does not rapidly transform these "foreign energies" (energies derived from food), it runs the risk of being overtaken by them. Foods will encumber the digestive tube, ferment, and putrefy, producing a quantity of poison.

The body is therefore constantly at work digesting the mass of food and drink we ingest, meal after meal, day after day. But when food intake is halted, this digestive energy can be directed toward other tasks. After digestion, the body's second most demanding task is elimination of toxins to avoid being poisoned. Generally speaking, elimination work is never done sufficiently, precisely because most available energy is applied to the digestive domain. Toxins, meanwhile, gradually increase in the body, compromising the internal cellular environment and paving the way for future disease.

During a fast—with suppression of digestive action—the body suddenly has much more energy at its disposal to purify tissues, cleanse blood, and eliminate wastes. These eliminations are evident in the increased work done by excretory organs. The liver filters blood more actively, neutralizes wastes and poisons, and expels them into the bile. The intestines disassimilate wastes, passing them through the intestinal mucosa along the entire extent of their surface (600 square meters; more than 700 square yards). The white, furred tongue of fasters is typical; it testifies to this dissassimilation (the waste products being expelled) at the upper, visible end of the digestive tract. The quantity of materials thus expelled outward by the body toward the intestinal excretory organ are such that even several weeks after the start of a fast (without any new intake from outside), the bowels can still expel fecal matter.

Because of the amount of waste the kidneys filter and release into urine, the urine becomes overfull and takes on a deep color and strong odor.

The excretory elements of the skin will also begin intense elimination of wastes accumulated in different areas of the body. Pimples, eczema, or itching may break out all over. Fasters sometimes sweat at night, and the skin might also ooze and feel clammy.

Strong expectorations can also manifest in the respiratory tract. The body will expel quantities of phlegm, causing fasters to sneeze and cough.

Identified by their location, two kinds of waste are distinguished: circulating and embedded. Those nearest the surface are the first to be eliminated. Toxins circulating in the blood or located in immediate proximity to capillaries can easily and quickly gain access to the bloodstream, where they are carried to excretory organs. Toxins already located in these organs are surface toxins as well, also included in the term *circulating toxins*. Opening, or decongesting, the excretory organs is all that is needed for these wastes to quickly exit the body.

Embedded wastes, on the other hand, are more difficult to eliminate. They have been driven deeper and deeper into the tissues during a period when toxins entered the body but the body could not expel them. Pushed farther down by subsequent waves of toxins, these wastes are firmly embedded in the tissues and difficult to dislodge. Merely reopening the excretory organs to the surface is insufficient to force them back up. They require more effective methods that function at the deepest levels.

Autolysis triggered by a fast is one of these methods. Toxins are broken down so they can be transported by cellular fluids into the circulatory system, where blood will then carry to the excretory organs those substances that cannot be reused. The longer the fast, the more these autolyzed wastes can make their way to the surface to be reused or eliminated from the body.

This clearing of toxins can be rough and intense, often experienced in the form of violent elimination crises—also known as *detoxification crises* and even *healing crises,* because they help restore the body to health by ridding it of wastes that encumber it.

Eliminatory Updating

During a fast, a process of eliminatory updating takes place, made possible by suppressed digestion, which puts more energy at the body's disposal to purify tissues, cleanse blood, and eliminate wastes.

HEALING CRISES

Healing crises occur during a fast primarily because the body has more energy to devote to elimination functions, and once circulating toxins have been eliminated, deep toxins have a free path to exit the body. Healing crises can manifest violently because excretory organs are forced to function at an accelerated pace to eliminate all the wastes coming their way. The body enters a state of crisis—crisis intended to protect the body by cleansing it.

Healing crises can take on diverse characteristics that resemble actual diseases: the skin may be covered with acne-like pimples, or it may ooze fluids as in certain forms of eczema; the bronchial tubes may become congested as in bronchitis; the nose may run as with a cold; and the joints may become inflamed as with rheumatism.

The similarity between a healing crisis and disease is not surprising. As we have seen, diseases are primarily healing crises triggered by the body as a means to cure itself.

Although at times spectacular, healing crises do not last long, ranging from a few hours to a few days in duration. Symptoms of the crisis rapidly disappear as the wastes that prompted them are expelled from the body.

Healing crises are beneficial, because they enable the body to clear significant quantities of toxin. It is important to recognize this, because manifestations of a crisis are sometimes severe and may prompt people who are insufficiently aware of them to abandon the cure.

Because they are salutary, these crises should not be repressed, but simply monitored to ensure that the excretory organs are not taxed beyond their capacities. Signs that the organs are overtaxed are eliminations that cause pain, inflammation, and blockage of the excretory organs.

Healing Crises

Healing crises are the result of the body's intensified internal cleansing. For this reason, they are also referred to as *cleansing crises* or *detoxification* crises.

FASTING AND ACIDITY

The problems that acidification* causes in the cellular environment are becoming more widely known. Excess acid irritates the organs, results in demineralization, and interferes with enzymatic activity. Numerous illnesses can result, including rheumatism, sciatica, tendinitis, eczema, constant fatigue, hair loss, nervousness, leg cramps, sensitive gums, osteoporosis, and depression. Yet one often hears it said that fasting is beneficial because it acidifies the blood. How is this possible? Isn't this a contradiction?

Among the various toxins, a critical role is played by toxic acids. This arises from the fact that modern diets are rich in acidifying foods (meats, fats, sugars, grain) and poor in alkalizing foods (salad greens, raw and cooked vegetables, and so forth). Base or alkaline foods are eaten in quantities too small to counterbalance and neutralize the high acid intake.

As a result of this dietary imbalance, the pH of internal cellular environments—a measure of their acidity or alkalinity—tends toward the acid.

As with other toxins, high acid levels are not well tolerated in the blood; they alter blood composition and compromise its function, disrupt mental processes, and even threaten the body's survival. To correct this imbalance, the body seeks to filter as much acid as possible through excretory organs that specialize in this task: the lungs, kidneys, and skin.

Too often, the body needs to eliminate more acid than the excretory organs can handle. Only one solution is available to deal with the excess acids: push them deeper into tissues, where they are more easily tolerated. This raises the overall

---

*See also by Christopher Vasey *The Acid-Alkaline Diet for Optimum Health,* Rochester, VT: Healing Arts Press, 2003, revised and expanded edition, 2006.

acid level of the internal cellular environment, but helps the blood retain its normal pH of 7.3, or it may even become very slightly more alkaline than usual.

This blood alkalization makes sense: it is a protective technique to prevent blood pH from falling into acidity. In fact, the slight increase in alkalinity means blood is now able to neutralize excess acids that threaten its normal pH. Furthermore, the extra alkaline substances help blood to neutralize acids pushed down into the internal cellular environment according to this formula: 1 alkaline substance + 1 acid substance = 1 neutral salt. The greater the acidification of the internal cellular environment, the greater the degree of alkalinity required in the blood. The pH values of blood are therefore opposite of those in the cellular environment.

But this involves only a tendency toward alkalization and not an actual increase in alkalization, which the blood could not tolerate any better than acidification. Blood pH tends to remain stable at a very slightly alkaline but almost neutral level. The blood's movement toward alkalosis, then, is not entirely proportional to the internal cellular environment's drift toward acidosis.

Now we can better understand why one might say a fast is beneficial because it "acidifies" the blood. In reality, blood has not become acidic: it becomes *less alkaline*—in other words, it has moved toward the acidic end of the pH scale only by becoming less alkaline. But because the blood pH reflects the opposite of the internal cellular environment, this means that the "acidification" of the blood takes place in tandem with a deacidification of the internal environment.

During a fast, the internal cellular environment—all the cells and fluids in which they are immersed—loses acids. Consequently, it recovers a normal pH. Tissues are cleared of acids that hinder cellular exchanges by interfering with the activity of enzymes, which are highly sensitive to changes in pH. Acid wastes also attack tissues and organs, causing lesions and mineral loss. Healing and health are thus promoted when the internal cellular environment regains its normal composition.

The level of acid elimination can be evaluated by observing urination. Normal urine has a pH level of 7.0 to 7.3. Any increase of the quantity of acids eliminated alters this pH. The more acids eliminated from tissues, the higher the acidity of urine.

pH Levels

The pH values of the blood are opposite those of the internal cellular environment. If the blood becomes slightly acidified (less alkaline) during a fast, it is because the internal environment is becoming less acidic.

During the course of a fast, then, urine typically increases in acidity as quantities of acid are expelled during eliminatory updating or a healing crisis. Acids are produced by autolysis as well, making the acidification of urine a normal response, and even beneficial, as it points to the internal cellular environment recovering its normal pH.

To facilitate understanding, one benefit of fasting can be understood not as acidifying the blood, but as deacidifying the internal cellular environment.

THE BENEFITS OF FASTING

During a fast, substances that are harmful to the body—wastes and diseased tissue—are destroyed and eliminated, whether by the normal purging function of excretory organs or through the heightened action of healing crises.

In the best cases, cleansing means the body's internal cellular environment has recovered its ideal composition: blood is purified, lymph is cleared, cells are immersed in fluids freed of poisons and toxins, and organs can once more function freely. Cleansing occurs no matter what disease (or diseases) the faster is coping with. This physical cleansing is the core benefit of fasting—the basis of a fast's therapeutic value. By cleaning the cellular environment, it removes the true, common cause of disease and sets the faster on the road to healing. This fact is apparent to those who understand the fundamental role played by the internal cellular environment in overall health. Those who consider illnesses a localized problem caused by specific afflictions will have trouble grasping the true therapeutic benefits of a well-managed fast.

Of course, the intensity of cleansing—whether or not it occurs in the deep tissues and whether or not it is complete—depends on the autolytic capacity of the faster's system, as well as on the length of the fast. Complete results are not obtained in every fast. In some cases, autolysis and eliminatory updating are insufficient to resolve the faster's health problem—as seen in the case of Brandt, who, despite numerous, lengthy fasts, failed to eliminate her tumor through autolysis alone.

In the course of searching for another regimen that could provoke and maintain autolysis intense enough to have done with her tumor, she discovered the virtues of the grape mono diet. The reasons why a mono diet succeeded when a stricter fasting regimen did not will be addressed later in the book.

3

Cleansing Enemas

Brandt enthusiastically recommended enemas every day during the fast and for the duration of the grape mono diet. Daily enemas are likely to be too much for our modern physiologies. Enemas should be repeated twice a week over a period of two to three weeks to achieve deep cleansing.

The value of this cleansing method becomes clear when one gains a better understanding of intestinal function.

Intestines are divided into two major parts:

- The small intestine, which is approximately 18 feet (5.5 meters) long and about 1 inch (2.5 centimeters) in diameter
- The large intestine or colon, about 5 feet (1.5 meters) long with a diameter that varies from 2 to 2.5 inches (5 to 6 centimeters)

The small intestine begins at the exit of the stomach and ends in the lower-left quadrant of the abdomen, where the colon begins, whose terminus is the anus.

Food digestion takes place in the small intestine, carried out by juices secreted by the intestine itself, as well as secretions provided by the liver and pancreas. During the process, foods are broken down into their component substances to be subsequently absorbed through the intestinal walls.

These walls consist of a single layer of extremely delicate cells, behind which blood capillaries are located. Crossing through the intestinal wall, nutrients enter the bloodstream, where they are carried to the liver by the portal vein. There, depending on the particular nutrient, the liver will use them as they are, transform them to a more usable form, or combine them with other substances.

Despite their delicacy, the intestinal mucous membranes function like an intelligent filter, allowing only those substances the body can use to pass through their net. But this holds true only as long as the membranes have not been damaged. Unfortunately, damage can occur from any number of common causes. If the walls suffer lesions, intestines can allow a variety of wastes and poisons to pass through to the blood. The liver can neutralize and eliminate toxins that are carried to it, but this ability diminishes when autointoxication is extended over time.

Overcome by waves of toxins arriving in a ceaseless stream, the liver eventually loses the ability to cope with them and passes them through to the body without neutralizing them. The contamination of blood and body tissues that results is, as we have seen, the source of disease. This fact inspires many medical practitioners to declare that "disease begins in the intestine."

Intestinal walls become porous and stop filtering properly for many reasons:

1. **Foods eaten can be natural irritants:** alcohol, excess caffeine, spices, sugars, and acids fall into this category. Foods may also contain chemical substances that are irritants: preservatives, food coloring, insecticides,

pesticides, and other pollutants. Medications and drugs can also irritate mucous membranes.

2. **Poor digestion deteriorates intestinal walls:** fermentation and putrefaction of the mass of food passing through the digestive tract produces quantities of aggressive substances like indoles and skatoles (active organic compounds) that can damage the membranes.

3. **Retaining fecal matter in the intestines too long damages membranes:** constipation prolongs the contact between mucous membranes and harmful wastes and toxins. In the case of chronic constipation, such material will adhere to intestinal walls in layers that can be over an inch to an inch and a half (3–4 centimeters) thick and tough (like rubber). These deposits become permanent irritants that interrupt the proper function of intestinal mucous membranes.

4. **A poor-quality diet or overeating alters the intestinal environment:** the wrong foods—as well as insufficient intestinal evacuations—will alter the intestinal milieu and bring about changes to the intestinal flora, microorganisms that normally live in the gut and assist with proper digestion. These microorganisms can become pathogenic germs when the intestinal milieu in which they work deteriorates.

Intestinal contents can also convert to a mass of putrefying and fermenting matter, teeming with germs and saturated in toxins. And this mass sits inside of us, separated from our internal environment by a fine mucous membrane no more than 25–30 thousandths of a millimeter thick! For any cure to be effective, this mass of poisons and waste must be eliminated from the body. Anti-symptomatic treatments may provide some relief, but they fail to address the root of the problem: diseases can be self-maintaining simply by virtue of the deplorable state of the intestines.

Enemas deal directly with the problem by cleansing and ridding the intestine of wastes. They work by introducing water into the intestine where it can liquefy fecal matter and facilitate its evacuation. Water dilutes this material, dislodges crusts that have attached to the intestinal walls, and carries toxins out of the body when the liquid is expelled.

Enemas imitate the body's natural defense system for getting rid of germs or poisons: diarrhea. Intestinal eliminations are complete during an occurrence of diarrhea because the contents are liquefied.

We should keep in mind that intestines are not merely tubes with smooth walls, but are tubes with countless folds and small projections (intestinal villi) among which wastes can hide. Only by promoting the passage of water through these folds can wastes be dislodged.

In practice, it is easy to see how this "emptying" of the intestines alters the course of a disease. Enemas act like the release of a clutch—fever falls, pain diminishes, and other problems recede. In this way, the patient conserves energy for other tasks—physical energy that previously went toward coping with the consequences of an intestine full of waste.

Enemas also free intestinal mucosa of crusts and adhered wastes, allowing the process of intestinal dissassimilation to resume working efficiently. In fact, the collected wastes lying stagnant in tissues surrounding the intestines can then cross through the intestinal mucosa to be eliminated with the stools. This process of disassimilating wastes, which takes place along the entire extent of the mucous membranes in the alimentary canal, is visible only when it occurs on the tongue. A white tongue and furry mouth are the signs of this elimination.

Enemas

The principle of enemas is the introduction of water into the intestines to liquefy fecal matter and facilitate its elimination.

Enemas are beneficial because they:
- Free the intestines of a mass of stagnating wastes
- Prevent fermentation and putrefaction
- Expel from the intestines poisons that are irritating and harsh on mucous membranes
- Encourage assimilation of nutrients and disassimilation of toxins by the intestinal mucosa

Applying enemas not only empties the intestines of collected waste, but also allows the mucous membranes along their entire surface to pass wastes through from the tissues. This represents more than 700 square yards (600 square meters) of disassimilation surface! It would be unfortunate to deprive the body of this important exit by neglecting to take the necessary enemas.

More information about the practice of using enemas can be found in chapter 7, beginning on page 85.

4

The Grape Mono Diet

After the initial stage of preparation—fasting and enemas—Brandt's regimen continues to the actual Grape Cure from which the practice takes its name. In this second stage, the fast is broken and only grapes are eaten. They are the exclusive item at every meal.

Because only one food is allowed, the regimen is called a mono diet—consisting of a single (mono) food. Mono diets can be fashioned around all kinds of foods. The basic principle is to select one and remain with it for the duration of the cure. The food can be eaten as often as one likes during the cure, at mealtimes and between—but always alone and never supplemented. The food must be a healthy choice so that benefits of the diet are not lost due to deficiencies in the food itself. A mono diet of eggs, meat, or chocolate, for instance, would soon cause digestive problems and the production of copious wastes. As a general rule, mono diets are practiced with grains, or with fruits and vegetables served raw, cooked, or in juice form. More information on foods suitable for mono diets will be discussed in The Mono Diet in Practice in chapter 7.

Mono diets are extremely strict regimens that bear a close resemblance to fasting, in that all foods have been removed except one. The effects of a mono diet are thus similar to those of a fast.

To be sure, substantial quantities of the chosen food—in this case grapes—can be consumed over the course of a day. However, as it only involves a single food, the digestive system's work is vastly simplified. There are no digestive conflicts as may occur when foods are mixed during the course of a normal meal, and digestion can proceed with ease. The nutritive substances consumed are rapidly absorbed, and the body enters a state similar to that of a fast.

THE BASIC VIRTUES OF THE MONO DIET

Because fasts and mono diets are so similar in practice, the same healing phenomena triggered by fasts are also triggered by mono diets. Autolysis, the updating of eliminations, and tissue regeneration all occur in mono diets. These healing reactions are somewhat less intense, as mono diets are less restrictive than fasts; nevertheless, the same bodily responses arise.

Autolysis is triggered as soon as the body needs nutritive substances that are not present—or are present only in limited quantity—in the food that is chosen for the diet. To continue functioning normally, the body draws nutrients from within itself by autolysis. This autolysis of tissues will continue for the duration of the cure. Diseased tissues and toxins are broken down and the internal cellular environment is cleansed, just as in a fast.

Eliminatory updating may also occur during a mono diet when the energy normally called on for digestion is sharply reduced. Purifying processes can then be activated to extract toxins from the tissues and carry them via the transport systems of blood and lymph to the excretory organs. In addition to this purification triggered by energy savings in digestion, specific purifying properties of the mono diet food are at work. For example, diuretic and laxative properties of the grape itself reinforce the purification properties of the diet.

Tissue regeneration also takes place due to cleansing that improves circulation and promotes efficient exchange of autolyzed substances, as well as by the intake of important nutrients contained in the selected food.

The fact that autolysis, eliminatory updating, and tissue regeneration take place at a slower pace is not necessarily a drawback. This should not prompt one to fast for longer periods rather than following a mono diet. As we shall see, mono diets have a number of advantages over fasts alone.

The first advantage is, in fact, that the cleansing processes do take place slowly. An abrupt, massive return of toxins is less likely, and the patient is spared the violent healing crises they can provoke. This is an advantage for the elderly, for those with diminished vitality, and for anyone suffering a major illness or severe autointoxication—those whose weakened bodies are less able to tolerate a violent elimination crisis. In fact, such individuals run the risk of an excretory organ becoming overworked or momentarily blocked under the avalanche of waste that can flood their system during a more severe fasting diet.

Heavy meat eaters, fans of large meals, as well as those whose bodies have been saturated with drugs or medications, are also more comfortable on a mono diet, for by choosing the less restrictive regimen, they are spared painful detoxification crises while still enjoying an opportunity to take an active role in their own health.

Another advantage of a less restrictive diet is that a level of physical function can be sustained, due to food intake. Some bodies are so worn out, they can no longer retain normal rhythms without external stimulation. For want of strength and internal tone, they need to be set in motion and maintained by stimuli derived from foods. This is a little like a person who drinks a lot of coffee and finds it difficult to wake up in the morning without it.

For people dependent on the stimulation provided by food, an overly restrictive diet like a fast will rob them of this critical aid. Their bodily functions will slow down, autolysis will not occur—or it will happen poorly at best—and eliminations will stop dead in their tracks. This kind of body functions in slow motion during a fast, but by maintaining food intake—if only one kind in a mono diet—this stimulation is sustained and so is physical function and the healing process.

This is what Brandt realized; this is why she opted for a mono diet as the foundation of her treatment, rather than fasting alone.

In her system, the purpose of fasting before beginning the grape mono diet is to trigger autolysis and cleansing by the drastic reduction of food intake for a short time. These processes, which will continue even when grapes are introduced, could not be activated so intensely by starting out immediately with the mono diet.

Another advantage of less restrictive diets, one not to be dismissed, is the psychological aspect. Some people are afraid of not eating. In fact, the tensions that result from this fear can block circulation and nerve impulses while interfering with organ function. By allowing one food that can be eaten at will, this fear dissipates and their bodies can function freely.

When organs are inactive, either because they are blocked by fear or they lack stimulation, they cannot perform their jobs adequately, which hampers the action of the cure.

Mono Diets

Like fasts, mono diets trigger autolysis of diseased tissue and toxins, eliminatory updating, and regeneration of tissues.

Advantages of the mono diet compared to fasting:
- Reduces the intensity of the healing crises
- Easier to do
- Removes the fear generated by not eating
- Stimulates and sustains body function with the help of a selected food

Although mono diets are proportionately less effective than fasts, their action is still remarkable. It resides—as with fasts—in autolysis, eliminatory updating, and physical regeneration.

The grape itself possesses wonderful detoxifying properties that combine with the three elements mentioned above; they do not replace them so much as complement them. Expecting to find the Grape Cure's benefits in the grape itself—as Brandt did—or expecting the full benefit in any single-food diet to lie in the food itself is a mistake.

Humans have become accustomed to the use of medicines and remedies, and they credit their cures to active substances in those remedies. In reviewing the results of the grape mono diet, there is therefore a temptation to attribute its virtues to some substance in the composition of the grape.

In fact, the effectiveness of mono diets does not depend on what is present (the grape, for example), but on what is not present (all other foods customarily eaten)—foods whose absence triggers autolysis.

The proof: eating quantities of grapes while continuing a normal diet does not bring about the same results as a diet of grapes alone.

One could also ask why, when interrupting a fast to begin

a restrictive regimen like the grape mono diet, the healing properties of the fast (autolysis) would not suddenly disappear only to be replaced by those of the grape. Autolysis, which is the most salutary effect of both fasts and diets, continues from the fast through the mono diet.

By absorbing only small quantities of grapes, the Grape Cure becomes very much like a fast and its intense autolytic processes are maintained.

Brandt seems to have been aware of this, because she wrote: "We have noted that the best results are obtained when the patients take only small quantities of grapes."

Based on these facts, good results could also be expected from mono diets based on foods other than grapes. In truth, wonderful results have been obtained with other mono diets, for both mild disorders and those as serious as cancer. The Breuss vegetable juice cure (celery, beet, potato, black radish) is a well-known example. The rice mono diet has been highly successful in macrobiotics. The legendary health of the people of Hunza in northern Pakistan is due in part to the mono diets of dried apricots and fasting they must follow at the end of each winter when their food stores are depleted. The mono diet of spinach alternating with white cheese was made famous by a woman—an American doctor—Degolière-Davenport who, after a serious illness, went on to live to the age of 120.

The Virtues of Mono Diets

The virtues of mono diets lie first in the processes of autolysis, eliminatory updating, and tissue regeneration. Secondary value is derived from the beneficial properties of the chosen food.

Many more examples exist. But by this diversity of foods that support successful mono diets, we must conclude that their principal virtue is not in their substance, as we have come to expect. It is in the dietary restriction itself, which triggers autolysis.

Having said that, grapes do have certain therapeutic properties. What are they?

PROPERTIES OF THE GRAPE

We shall first look at the medicinal properties of the grape, then its nutritional properties.

The Medicinal Properties of the Grape

Beyond its role in the cure itself, the grape is primarily recommended for its detoxifying properties—in other words, for its ability to encourage elimination of toxins by stimulating the excretory organs. In fact, the grape encourages the work of the main excretory organs.

DIURETIC ACTION

Grape consumption spurs the kidneys to filter more wastes, causing diuresis (increased excretion of urine). The increase in urine volume offers greater support for the transfer of toxins outside the body. This ensures that toxins filtered out of the blood will be eliminated from the body and will not remain to clog the renal filter.

Grapes are customarily recommended for patients who retain water (edema) and those suffering from kidney ailments (renal insufficiency, kidney stones, uremia, and even nephritis), as well as for disorders caused by renal insufficiency such as gout and rheumatism.

The grape's diuretic action is seen in the increased concentration of wastes in the urine, from which it takes on a darker color and stronger odor.

HEPATIC ACTION

Grapes are a stimulant and decongestant for the liver as well. By helping the liver to perform, grapes assist it in clearing impurities that stagnate in its tissue. Once clear, the liver is more efficient at filtering wastes brought to it by the blood and drawn from the depths of tissue.

The antitoxic function of the liver is also enhanced, allowing it to more effectively neutralize and destroy poisons, toxic metals, medications, drugs, products of pollution, carcinogenic substances, and cancerous cells. The fact that the grape is recommended in cases of poisoning is sufficient evidence of its action on the liver.

The grape exerts a positive effect on the gallbladder, emptying this pouch that receives bile sent its way by the liver. The gallbladder is also full of wastes the liver has filtered. Emptying the gallbladder encourages digestion and rapid intestinal transit and fights against fermentation and putrefaction, which are large producers of gas and toxins.

INTESTINAL ACTION

Grapes are a laxative, which means they gently stimulate intestinal transit and evacuation. Like all roughage consisting of plant fiber, grape skin and seeds carry wastes out of the body. Brandt points out that the seeds and skins act like brooms, peeling off the crust that covers the intestinal walls and sweeping it to the outside.

Good eliminations are fundamental for health. Not only are the intestines, because of their length, the excretory organ that can hold the largest mass of waste; what's more, they receive the toxins released in secretions from all the digestive glands: liver bile, saliva from the salivary glands, and so on. The intestines are also a site of assimilation, primarily of nutritive substances, but they also absorb toxins if these latter have damaged the intestinal mucosa, hampering its filtering capacity.

The grape exerts an "anti-putrefaction" effect on the contents of the intestines, thus reducing the production of poisons that are created by putrefaction and fermentation of the alimentary bolus (the mass of food being digested).

For some, however, this laxative effect does not occur. To the contrary, grapes cause constipation in some individuals. This is because grapes contain tannins, whose astringent properties cause the intestines to "tighten." In these cases, Brandt recommends eating only the fruit pulp, as the tannins are found primarily in the skin and seeds.

As we have seen, because of its purifying and detoxifying properties, the grape directly stimulates the activity of the excretory organs and sustains their function throughout the duration of the mono diet, something that does not occur during a fast. In a fast, the body itself has to stimulate the excretory organs. In a Grape Cure, the stimulation is provided by an external source: the grape. This clearly shows why Brandt believed the mono diet to be more detoxifying than a fast.

"The fast," she wrote, "only eliminates a portion of the inorganic deposits that are often the cause of a disease. This is perhaps why cancer cannot be cured by the fast alone. So fast, but complete the process with purification."

This purification that Brandt is alluding to is the grape mono diet.

The Nutritional Properties of the Grape

The principal constituent elements of the grape are provided in the table below (based on 100 grams of grapes, or approximately 1/4 pound).

The figures show that grapes are rich in carbohydrates,

which are energy foods for the body, and in minerals, which are building blocks for tissues. While the protein content is slight, it exists nevertheless. Although deficient in vitamins D, E, and F, grapes contain varying degrees of other vitamins and trace elements.

THE CONSTITUENT ELEMENTS OF THE GRAPE
Sample size: 100 grams

Calories	77
Water	81.3 g
Carbohydrates	16.6 g
Lipids	0.7 g
Proteins	0.9 g
Calcium	19.0 mg
Chlorine	2.0 mg
Copper	0.1 mg
Iodine	0.002 mg
Iron	0.45 mg
Magnesium	9.0 mg
Phosphorus	21.0 mg
Potassium	224.0 mg
Sodium	2.0 mg
Sulfur	9.0 mg
Zinc	0.1 mg
Vitamin A	0.024 mg
Vitamin B_1	0.05 mg
Vitamin B_2	0.02 mg
Vitamin B_2	0.3 mg
Vitamin B_5	0.08 mg
Vitamin B_6	0.09 mg
Vitamin C	5.0 mg

To explain the virtues of the Grape Cure, we could choose to address one by one the vitamins grapes contain, each trace element, and the individual minerals to demonstrate that thanks to:

- Vitamin A, grapes maintain tissue nutrition and encourage the regeneration of tissues
- Vitamin B₁ encourages the absorption of oxygen and thereby the oxidation of wastes
- Magnesium fights the development of tumors

But we can summarize by saying that the numerous vitamins and trace elements found in grapes encourage the balanced functioning of the body through their stimulating effect on enzymes. As we have seen, enzymes work properly only in the presence of sufficient vitamins and trace elements, and enzymes play the principal role in the phenomenon of—autolysis.

DOES THE GRAPE CURE CAUSE WEIGHT LOSS?

The Grape Cure can remove toxins from the body and heal it of numerous diseases, but is it capable of getting rid of extra pounds?

For a regimen to cause weight loss, it must be restrictive enough to trigger autolysis. In fact, it is due to autolysis that fats are broken down and weight loss occurs. The body will draw from its reserves—and its fat deposits—only if normal nutritional needs are not being met through food intake. Only when it is deprived of essential elements (proteins, carbohydrates, vitamins . . .) does the body draw out the necessary substances through autolysis. As we have seen, autolysis operates intelligently and first attacks nonessential tissue, among which are fat accumulations.

Is the Grape Cure sufficiently restrictive to trigger this weight-loss process? Grapes are rich primarily in vitamins and minerals. They contain only 17 grams of sugar for every 100 grams of grapes (approximately 1/4 pound), and negligible amounts of fat bodies. Their caloric value is 77 calories per 100 grams. Consumption of 1 kilogram of grapes per day (a little over 2 pounds) represents an intake of only 770 calories. The normal daily caloric intake is considered 2,400 calories, but in practice people in the United States consume closer to 3,700 calories. We are justified, then, in saying that the Grape Cure is a sufficiently restrictive diet to cause weight loss.

In her book, Brandt mentions that weight loss is a natural consequence of the cure. In her descriptions of case histories, she points to the large weight losses experienced by some of her patients. Experience garnered over the years indicates that numerous people return to their ideal weight due to this cure. In short, it can be used as a diet to shed pounds.

Unlike other cures, the Grape Cure is easy to follow. On the one hand, the chosen food has a pleasant taste even over the long term, as contrasted to high-protein regimens, for example, which rapidly grow tiresome. On the other hand, the grape's eliminatory properties allow toxins to exit the body as well as fat.

On its own, the weight-loss process frees quantities of toxins, because some toxins are liposoluble and will therefore specifically accumulate in fatty tissues. When the tissues are autolyzed, the toxins they contain will also leave the body. It is therefore imperative, during any weight-loss regimen, to burn off fat and encourage the toxins to evacuate—two processes the Grape Cure encourages perfectly.

Weight Loss

The Grape Cure can cause weight loss by triggering autolysis. Weight loss is also encouraged by the eliminatory properties of the grape.

As in all food diets, loss of weight can be substantial during the first two or three days—from 2 to 5 pounds—then sharply reduces to a point as few as 2 to 5 ounces a day. This daily loss continues to shrink, moreover, as the days go on.

The large losses during the first few days are not loss of actual body weight; they are due to evacuation of fecal matter held in the intestines and elimination of water retained in the tissues. True weight loss starts with autolysis, after several days on the cure. It begins with the loss of several ounces but quickly drops as the body seeks to conserve its resources: it doesn't know how long the cure will go on! If reserves are drawn on at the rate seen on the first days of the cure (several ounces), they would be rapidly exhausted, followed by death by starvation. The body normally seeks to slow autolysis as much as possible, so reserves will last longer—to the great despair of people hoping to lose weight.

To be effective, the weight-loss regimen must be sustained for a long enough time, something that is both possible and pleasant to do with a grape diet. The diet should not be continued for longer than two weeks, but can be repeated after a monthlong break.

A SUMMARY OF THE BENEFICIAL EFFECTS OF THE GRAPE CURE

The fast that Brandt recommends for the start of her cure not only allows the body to cleanse itself; it also fully triggers the autolysis process. By introducing a regimen as light as the grape mono diet, autolysis continues uninterrupted. Even more, physical functioning is sustained and autolysis is reinforced by the trace elements and vitamins contained in grapes.

Why the Grape Cure Is Effective

Medicinal properties of the Grape Cure:

- Eliminatory updating
- Tissue regeneration
- Diuretic
- Hepatic and biliary
- Laxative

Nutritional properties of the grape:

- Richness of vitamins and trace elements
- Stimulates enzymatic activity, thus autolysis

5

The Raw Food Diet

Several stages of Brandt's cure consist of an exclusively raw food diet. After the first-stage fast, the second stage is the grape mono diet. In the third stage, the exclusive diet of grapes is supplemented with other raw foods: various fruits, tomatoes, curdled milk, fromage blanc, and yogurt. The fourth stage—called the raw food stage—increases dietary choices to include nuts, eggs, butter, honey, and olive oil.

Brandt considered a raw food diet (crudivorism) best. She emphasized that, for people who are ill, remaining at the raw food stage is preferable to progressing to stage five, which includes cooked foods like potatoes, grains, bread, pasta, and some fish (but no meat). Stage five is offered only to those who, for one reason or another, cannot remain on raw foods exclusively. The fifth stage also comes with a warning that former health problems could reappear, provoked by a resumption of cooked foods in the diet.

Incontestably, crudivorism is beneficial. Just what are the benefits of raw food, and what harm does cooking do?

THE HARMFUL EFFECTS OF COOKING

One initial observation must come forward: cooking alters the vitality of food substantially. Plant a seed of raw wheat— it will germinate, sprout, and create a head full of grain. Plant a seed of cooked wheat—nothing happens; it will not sprout.

During cooking, the most valuable nutritional substances are altered. At 140°F (60°C), vitamins are destroyed; between 104°F (40°C) and 167°F (75°C), enzymes and hormones degrade; around 194°F (90°C), aromas disappear; and at 212°F (100°C), minerals will undergo molecular changes that make them more difficult for the body to use (that is, they lose the characteristic of more dynamic minerals, given life by the plant).

Another drawback of cooking is that it encourages mixing numerous foods at one meal, even in one dish: sauce with meat juices, flour, butter, or fat . . . or pastry with grains, fruits, eggs, sugar, oil, honey . . .

This blending has a disastrous effect on digestion. Each food, when it enters the digestive tube, prompts the secretion of specific digestive juices to process it. The more different foods are contained in one meal, the more the digestive organs (liver, stomach, pancreas, and so forth) will receive conflicting orders for the secretions they should release, and the more the digestive juices will be at odds with each other. In fact, certain digestive juices—for example, those of the stomach—are active only in an acid environment. If foods requiring alkaline secretions are eaten at the same time, they will render the stomach's environment less acidic. The gastric juices will be less effective—even unable to function—depending on the proportion of acid and alkaline substances introduced into the stomach. The result of these antagonisms is poorly digested food that ferments or putrefies; large amounts of toxins and poisons ensue, which alter intestinal flora and increase its pathogenic elements. These poisons irritate and damage intestinal mucosa, and they exhaust the liver, which receives them to be neutralized.

Separating those foods whose digestion requirements are at odds is therefore recommended, particularly for people with insufficient digestive capacity. Some individuals do not have enough digestive strength to process foods normally, no matter how they combine them. Without expressly mentioning it, the diet in Brandt's cure respects the major separate food groups, to the benefit of those who must deal with this insufficiency.

Cooking has another drawback. It encourages overeating. A person cannot eat as much raw food as cooked food; raw foods (vegetables, fruits, nuts, and so on) demand a greater effort to chew. Cooked food is also generally soft and can often be swallowed with almost no chewing required. The disadvantages of this are threefold: not only can a person eat too much; also, food that is insufficiently chewed reaches the digestive tract in larger pieces. It is consequently more difficult for the digestive enzymes to attack. Also, these foods have less exposure to saliva and are less saturated with the digestive juices that originate in the mouth. The beneficial effects of proper chewing were demonstrated by Horace Fletcher (1849–1919), an American naturopath, who cured many of his patients simply by having them chew their food for a full minute—"in order to make something solid into a liquid"—and this in the absence of any change to their regular diet![1]

On the other hand, cooking food has some advantages. It allows the intake of warmth—not a negligible quality for weakened individuals. Cooking reduces the harshness of fiber for those suffering from colitis, and it sparks the transformation of starches into carbohydrates, which are easier to digest. Cooking has also expanded the human diet, thereby enabling us to confront rigorous climates. In certain regions of the world, during winter, eating only raw foods is not possible.

While eating some cooked foods is not a bad thing, eating exclusively cooked foods is; in the latter case, the foods are often nearly devoid of their vitamins, which are destroyed during cooking.

Harmful Effects of Cooking

- Destroys the life of the food
- Encourages mixing of many foods
- Encourages overeating
- Reduces chewing time

Advantages of Cooking

- Brings in energy in the form of heat
- Reduces the harshness of fibers
- Facilitates the digestion of starches
- Permits the consumption of grains, potatoes, and so forth

THE BENEFITS OF A RAW FOOD DIET

The first advantage of a raw food diet is the elimination of foods that are generally eaten cooked—like meat, fish, pasta, and foods made with these products. This represents a reduction in the amount that will be eaten (true for all diets), but more importantly, the foods that are removed are the highest producers of toxins. By not eating them, the individual's body is relieved of a major source of waste.

Raw foods, on the other hand, are rich in vitamins and trace elements, whose function is to stimulate and enable the enzymatic activity on which all vital processes depend. By eating regular and generous portions of raw food, one consumes large quantities of enzyme activators. Due to this intake, body functions that were dulled by toxins and deficiencies are put back to work. The cells are reactivated to perform functions that were interrupted. The tissues "start breathing" again, wastes are burned off and eliminated, and the body's internal cellular environment purifies and regenerates itself.

Raw foods introduce not only enzyme activators, but also enzymes contained in the foods themselves. Every animal and plant body contains enzymes it needs to sustain life. They are available to the plant or animal for its own biochemical requirements.

When they enter our bodies, they now are available for our use. This constitutes an invaluable resource for a diseased body in which enzymatic activities are at their lowest ebb. The external supply of enzymes that can be consumed in raw foods increases the enzymatic capital of the individual suffering from illness; these enzymes can relaunch his metabolism and the healing process.

For people coping with disease, eating raw foods triggers an interior response like the effect of a cool breeze on embers that are in danger of going out—or like a water current reaching the hollow bed of a dry river. Crudivorism is essential for certain patients, enabling their bodies to begin functioning properly again. Brandt included the raw diet as a crucial part of her cure, making it an important element in the healing process for those who followed her regimen.

The benefits of a raw food diet, however, should not blind us to the fact that it is a *therapeutic diet,* and it cannot be continued indefinitely and exclusively. Serious nutrient deficiencies and a loss of vitality are common problems that can arise. In fact, on a strict raw food diet, protein intake is severely limited, as meat, fish, eggs, and dairy products are almost totally excluded. In addition, increased consumption of fruits, required by the elimination of other carbohydrate sources (grains, pastas, bread, cereals, potatoes), will tip the acid balance of the internal cellular environment and strip tissues of their mineral content.

Benefits of a Raw Food Diet

- Respects the "life" energy of foods (vitamins)
- Represents an intake of enzyme stimulants (vitamins, trace elements)
- Brings in enzymes

Problems with a Raw Food Diet

- Foods eaten bring in no heat
- Represents a severe reduction of proteins
- Causes acidification by an excess of fruits
- Causes irritation of the intestinal mucous membranes with excessive fiber content because raw fibers are much harsher than cooked fibers
- Limits nutritional choices and cannot be adhered to in climates where fresh foods are unavailable in winter

---

One must, therefore, exercise extreme care on an exclusively raw food diet. While it can be a beneficial therapeutic regimen over the short term, it must be practiced with restraint over the long term (when followed as a daily regimen). The best option is, once illness is cured, combine cooked food with a generous helping of raw vegetables.

6

Indications and Contraindications of the Grape Mono Diet

Diets in general, and the Grape Cure in particular, appear to be universally helpful and harmless. In practice, this may not be so. Regimens, diets, and fasts *are beneficial only for the specific conditions they aim to correct.* Countless patients and well-meaning individuals have learned this difficult truth—diets can improve health or they can destroy it. No one diet is "good for everyone." Every regimen—every diet—has its own characteristics and, consequently, its own indications and contraindications.

Patients have their own particular temperament, physical idiosyncrasies, and disorders, and each patient must choose a diet in accord with those characteristics to realize the benefits they hope for.

The Grape Cure—particularly the grape mono diet—has its own indications and contraindications. Of paramount importance, understanding these principles at the outset will spare patients from making the wrong choice.

The grape mono diet has two major contraindications: the first is a disproportionate physiological sensitivity to acids;

the second is failure to understand the nature of the healing crises triggered by the cure.

We shall take up each of these in turn here, but an extra note of caution is warranted on the issue of healing crises: During the course of this cure, various detoxification crises will almost certainly occur. Initially, they are beneficial; after a time, they can be harmful. The patient must learn to recognize when this dividing line is reached and stop the cure. An understanding of the different phases of a diet (discussed beginning on page 75) is key in determining this point. See also Destructive Healing Crises on page 77 and Urgent Signs to Stop Fasting on page 93.

PHYSICAL SENSITIVITY TO ACIDS

Foods contain varying proportions of acid and alkaline substances (the latter are known also as *bases*). Many acid foods can be directly identified by their sharp taste: grapefruit, vinegar, and yogurt, for example. Other foods are not acid in themselves, but they acidify the body when digested or during the course of transformations they undergo at the cellular level. Included among these acidifying foods are meats, grains, white sugar, beans, fats, coffee, and wine.

Other foods contain primarily base substances and are known as alkalizing foods: vegetables, potatoes, bananas, and almonds, for instance.

We all naturally eat foods that are acid, acidifying, and alkalizing. But depending on how much of each food group we ingest, the body can become acidified—a little, a lot, or not at all.

To function properly, the human body should maintain a pH of 7.3. The pH is a scale used to measure the acidity or alkalinity of a substance. The scale ranges from 0 to 14, with 0 indicating absolute acidity and 14 absolute alkalinity. The blood's pH of 7.3 is therefore nearly neutral, but tipping toward alkaline.

The human body seeks a stable pH, but the level is constantly modified by dietary factors as well as by stress, vitamin deficiencies, physical activity, tissue oxygenation, and more. Lifestyle therefore exerts a strong influence on pH. But overly large variations in the acid/alkaline balance will cause illness.

All vital processes both within and around the cells occur by virtue of enzymatic activity. This activity relies on the pH of the immediate cellular environment. In other words, each enzyme has an ideal pH for optimal performance. If pH is altered, an enzyme's activity is hampered, slows down, or can cease entirely. Illness and even death may result.

The body therefore strives to maintain pH as close to the ideal as possible. The three primary processes used to achieve this are:

1. **Directly neutralizing food acids with alkaline substances carried in by the same foods.** One acid and one base (alkaline substance) equal one neutral salt. For this to work, however, foods must contain enough of the required substances. In addition, only those acids present in the digestive tract will be neutralized in this way, not those produced in tissues at the cellular level.

2. **Using oxidation to neutralize acid in tissues.** Oxidation transforms acids into nonacidic substances and into wastes for elimination—for instance, carbon dioxide (CO_2) and water, which are expelled by the lungs and kidneys. Sufficient oxygen, vitamins, and trace elements are required for oxidation to occur.

3. **Employing the anti-acid defense system known as "buffering power."** This method neutralizes acids by

deacidifying them (buffering them) with alkaline minerals drawn out of the tissues themselves (instead of from food, as in the first method). All tissues are subject to this extraction—bone, nail, skin, cellular fluid, and so on. Most affected are tissues rich in alkaline minerals such as calcium, magnesium, potassium, iron, and zinc.

Buffering is integral to the body's function and does not cause serious problems unless called upon too often or too heavily. But if day after day—or several times a day—the body resorts to its buffer system, alkaline reserves will be depleted. Prolonged theft of these minerals will cause damage, as they are pillaged not from a special reserve, but from the tissues themselves. The result is demineralization of the body. Initially, this is betrayed by minor symptoms like hair loss, fragile nails, less tone, dry and chapped skin and lips, dental caries, cold sores, rectal and urinary burning, colds and chronic sinusitis, and insomnia. These may be followed by more serious disorders and lesions including eczema, pulmonary problems, depression, rheumatism, sciatica, headaches, irritability and increased nervous sensitivity, low blood pressure, and immune deficiencies.

As a general rule, people with a robust, expansive, ruddy, congestive, hot temperament generally have a high capacity for oxidizing acids and good mineral reserves to buffer them, because their bones have a higher concentration of minerals. Conversely, people with a nervous, withdrawn, cold, phlegmatic temperament oxidize acids poorly, and have smaller mineral reserves available to buffer the acids.

Of the two types, the first processes acids well; such people neutralize acids easily and even transform them into alkaline minerals using their powerful oxidizing capacity. This can be discerned in such individuals by increased alkalization of their urine following consumption of acidic foods like lemons, for example.

The second group metabolizes acids poorly. By ingesting acidic foods too often or in large quantities, they accumulate acids that attack their tissues, forcing alkaline minerals out of them. Furthermore, they are deficient at oxidizing these acids and transforming them to alkaline substances. Unlike the preceding group, their urine shows a rise in acidity when they eat acid foods.

We begin to see the danger here of trying to determine the alkalizing effect of a diet by analyzing the food content alone, or by measuring its effect on urine. Any attempt to determine the impact of a diet on a specific individual must consider also the metabolic capacity of that person's body to process the acids it ingests.

In fact, if grapes are considered an alkalizing influence, it is because they contain more alkaline minerals (potassium, sodium, calcium, magnesium, iron) than acid minerals (phosphorus, sulfur, chlorine). However, in addition to minerals, grapes contain acids that must be neutralized as well, and these must enter into any calculations. Do grapes contain enough alkaline minerals to neutralize all the acids?

The urinary pH test is meant to answer this question. This test is easy to perform, requiring only litmus paper or pH Test Strips, which are more accurate and easier to read. (See the resources section on page 160 for information on ordering pH Test Strips.) To perform the test, hold a strip in the flow of urine for a second or two, just long enough to moisten it. The acid of the urine reacts with the paper, causing it to change color. By matching the paper with the indicator scale on the color chart, the urine's pH is obtained. A pH of 7.0 is neutral, 6.5 and lower is acid, and 7.5 and above is alkaline.

The concept underpinning this test is the belief that if the body absorbs excess alkaline or acid substances, it will expel them in the urine, where they can be measured. Consequently, if urine becomes more alkaline (a pH higher than 7.3) after eating, the supposition is that the food provides more alkaline minerals than the body needs and it allows the excess to be expelled. Conversely, urine supposedly becomes more acidic when food brings in too much acid and the excess is expelled.

Because the consumption of fruit generally causes an alkaline urine pH, it is mistakenly believed that fruits are alkalizing—mistakenly, because this urinary pH reveals the alkalinity of the urine and not that of body tissues.

As observed by Dr. Paul Carton, urine can be alkaline following the consumption of acid foods for two very different reasons: because the acids were oxidized and gave off numerous alkaline substances or because the body surrendered alkaline substances in an attempt to neutralize the acids.[1] In the first case, the increase in alkaline pH is a healthy response, corresponding to a real gain in alkaline substances in the body. In the second case, the presence of alkaline substances in urine betrays a loss of alkalizing minerals from the tissues as they attempted to neutralize acids. In the first case there is a gain, a replenishment of alkaline minerals, and increased health. In the second, there is a loss, a depletion of mineral content, and a reduction in health.

People who are sensitive to acids, for whom the grape mono diet is contraindicated, are in this second group. The Grape Cure diet is especially dangerous for them, as it will deplete their mineral content. Grapes—like all other fruits—contain acids, in lower concentration than many other fruits, but still present in sufficient quantity to increase the acid content of anyone on the mono diet who eats just this one food.

Acid Sensitivity and the Grape Cure: Is the Cure Suitable for You?

The Grape Cure will be favorable for you if you are not sensitive to acids, meaning:

- You are an expansive, ruddy, congestive type who is resistant to cold and fatigue
- You do not suffer from acidification problems
- Your urinary pH is normally 7.0 or higher
- A generous consumption of fruits will:
  - alkalize your urine
  - increase your vitality
  - banish health problems

The Grape Cure is contraindicated for you if you are sensitive to acids, meaning:

- You are a withdrawn, rather thin, pale, nervous type who tires quickly
- You are suffering or have suffered from various acidification problems
- Your urinary pH is acid: 6.5 or lower
- Your urine pH is alkaline and you have problems with acidification
- A generous consumption of fruits will:
  - acidify your urine
  - reduce your vitality
  - cause the appearance of new disorders and increase those that already exist

---

The Grape Cure is equally as beneficial for those individuals who metabolize acids well (cleansing them of toxins and restoring mineral balance) as it is contraindicated and dangerous for people who are sensitive to acids.

HEALING CRISES

People often boast of the benefits of the Grape Cure that restored them to health, while others report bitterly that this same cure destroyed their health. And those who suffered are not only people who are sensitive to acids! A change of health status can also develop as a consequence of the detoxification crises (healing crises) triggered by the cure.

To understand why healing crises can help in some cases and harm in others, we need to understand, phase by phase, the process that occurs during diets in general, including in the Grape Cure.

The Phases of a Diet

Consider the case of Mr. X.

Phase I. Mr. X overeats and rarely does any physical exercise. He burns off what he eats inefficiently and has overloaded his body with toxins. His vital force is insufficient to meet the demands of his lifestyle. Illnesses related to this overloading appear: headaches, inflammation of the respiratory tract, and arthritic pains.

Phase II. Aware of his condition and the health problems engendered, Mr. X undertakes a diet. The reduction in food intake means his body does less work to digest the food. This means Mr. X's vital force is now more than he needs to complete any other work he must do. In reality, the strength of this force has remained the same, but his energy seems greater because his body's workload has been reduced. His eliminatory organs are the first to benefit from this restoration of available energy and they increase their activity.

Phase III. The diet has lasted long enough for his body to eliminate most of the wastes it has stored up; Mr. X is relieved of toxins. His health problems have disappeared due to this cleansing, prompted by the diet cure. The intake of nutrients provided by the diet—or his physical reserves, in the event of a fast—are still sufficient to meet the needs of his body with its reduced workload (only minimal digestive and eliminatory work to do). Mr. X therefore feels a renewed sense of well-being. He feels light, in top form, and clear-headed. In fact, the vital forces and the diet are well balanced with his body's needs.

Phase IV. If Mr. X continues the regimen over the long term, his nutritive reserves (in the case of a fast) or food intake (with diets) will eventually become insufficient to support normal organ function. The physical slowdown that results will provoke an increase in waste production, as foods are poorly transformed and poorly eliminated. The toxins released by cellular activity will again exceed his body's capacity to eliminate them, as his energy will again subside.

Phase V. If the cure is not ended now, Mr. X's body, deprived of essential nutrients (vitamins, trace elements, minerals, amino acids, and so forth), will become severely deficient. Physical functions will continue to slow down or come to a halt, and lesions will appear (osteoporosis, chapped skin, and the like). These additional disorders appear, no longer caused by excess but instead by deficiency.

Phase VI. If the cure were to continue beyond this point, Mr. X. would risk starvation and death.

Beneficial Healing Crises

Beneficial crises take place during phase II, when the vital force is strong enough to actively cleanse the body. The crises are intense but generally of short duration, lasting from several hours to one or two days. They usually resemble disorders from which the patient has suffered in the past. In fact, these healing crises are a continuation of past efforts, however incomplete, to rid the body of toxins encumbering its internal cellular environment. These efforts were never completed, perhaps for lack of energy, or they may have been aborted by anti-symptomatic medications.

Healing crises are desirable, helping the body to rid itself of toxin surpluses. Although they're disagreeable to experience, after a crisis has passed, the patient feels much better.

Several healing crises can follow in succession—interspersed by calmer periods—each taking a different form (headaches, pimple outbreaks, feelings of heaviness, fatigue, or reactivations of old disorders), as the layers of waste become "unglued" from the deeper tissues and seek exit from the body.

The State of Well-Being

When the bulk of wastes have been eliminated, a period of well-being sets in (phase III). This is the result of achieving a new balance in the various forces present. *This stage must not be mistaken for balanced health that can be maintained permanently.* In reality, this is not balanced health, nor can it be maintained in this fashion over time. It is a result of the diet—not a normal routine that can be continued for years, but rather a restrictive therapeutic regimen that, precisely because of its therapeutic and restrictive nature, should not be continued indefinitely. This is an unstable, temporary balance brought about by the cure. It will come to an end, to be followed by phase IV if the cure is continued or by a second state of balance when eating is resumed.

Destructive Healing Crises

When the cure has reached phase III of well-being, the patient has exhausted the effects of the diet for the time being. The regimen must be stopped at this point by gradually resuming a normal, balanced diet, adapted to the physical capacities of the dieter over the long term. Therapy is replaced by good health practice.

Unfortunately, people often remain on the therapeutic diet, believing it to be an optimum regimen because it made them feel so good for a short time. However, because it is a diet that lacks several important nutrients, their bodies will function poorly (phases IV and V). They may seek to recapture the well-being they experienced in phase III by continuing or even increasing the restriction of the diet.

As body functions slow down and organs cannot perform their jobs, digestion degrades, nutritive substances are not properly broken down, and eliminations are reduced. Wastes accumulate, increased by a weakened metabolism. The internal cellular environment builds up waste deposits, the blood thickens, and the organs become congested, prompting a reappearance of illnesses spawned by this buildup. The individual following the cure may view this condition from a mistaken perspective and hail the symptoms as a healing crisis. But these symptoms are not at all like healing crises that took place in phase II; they are health disorders caused by excess wastes clogging tissues—back to phase I.

Thinking of them as healing crises is a mistake; they are not the result of intense efforts to rid the body of toxins (as the vital force is quite diminished and not capable of this); they result from the tissue congestion that happens when *wastes exceed the body's elimination capacity!* Rather than healing, they are destructive crises. Their characteristics are the opposite of those in phase II; the manifestations of this congestion are not short and intense; they are weak and long lasting. They persist and get worse if the cure is continued.

If the individual stubbornly continues on this course on the premise that a new healing crisis will bring on a new phase of well-being, he or she will exhaust all strength reserves and more deficiencies will appear. A person on this path—whether through stubbornness or poor guidance—can destroy good health (phase VI).

> ### Beneficial or Destructive?
>
> Beneficial healing crises are short, followed by improvements in health disorders and a general sense of well-being. The cure can be continued.
>
> Harmful healing crises, or "false" crises, repeat or persist for more than a day or two. They bring about a reduction of vitality and are not followed by improvements in health disorders. Stop the cure.

HOW LONG SHOULD THE DIET BE CONTINUED?

Deciding how long a diet should last is complicated further: some individuals, even before they start the cure, can already be in phase IV (congestion due to devitalization) or in phase V (congestion due to deficiencies). This often becomes apparent when a patient suffering from devitalization and deficiencies embarks on an overly strict and rigorous cure. The weak nutritive intake—or the absence of any nutrient intake, in the event of a fast—taxes their scant resources. They rapidly find themselves suffering from malnutrition, their bodies incapable of functioning correctly. For people who metabolize acids poorly, a fruit cure (lemon, grape) or a fruitarian diet has this effect. These diets will propel these individuals directly to phase IV or V, with subsequent loss of vitality and onset of malnutrition.

In the cases cited above, the question is not "When should I stop the diet?" but "What diet should I choose?" Such individuals should not begin a restrictive diet; they should opt immediately for a revitalizing regimen—which is to say, a balanced diet rich in a variety of nutrients—to help them regain their energy and correct their deficiencies. Paradoxically, such a diet can still help them clear toxins by promoting improved function so the body can break down and eliminate wastes that are burdening it. Logically, the visceral organs can fail to perform their tasks—burdening the internal cellular environment with an excess of waste—as much by overexertion and overeating as by loss of vitality and nutritive deficiencies.

Unfortunately, no absolute rule will allow one to determine with certainty whether an individual following a cure is experiencing a phase II healing crisis (and thereby may continue the cure) or has reached phase IV or V, the stages of false crises. To determine how long a diet should last, one must consider not only the elements of the diet itself, but also the patient's lifestyle, the kind of food eaten prior to the cure, past illnesses, and any physical weaknesses. By careful observation of these factors, the level of waste congestion and the body's potential for clearing these wastes can be ascertained. Keeping these factors in mind while observing the cure's progress, one can identify which phase of the cure the patient is experiencing.

If doubts persist, one should not hesitate to resume a normal diet to observe how the body copes. If the person following the cure is in phase IV or V, the crisis will end; vitality will return, and the general condition will improve. If the individual is going through phase II of the cure, a resumption of regular eating habits will bring no relief. If this is the case, the individual should return to the diet.

In case of doubt, Hippocrates recommended alternating the use of opposing therapeutic agents, thereby banishing narrow-minded and sectarian tendencies and appealing to vigilance and an open mind. He wrote:

Man's regimen is designed for the dry to be moistened, the wet be dried, that things be divided, separated, and brought together so that health is procured by a host of contrary things. . . . When the strict diet causes harm, one must change to a nourishing regimen and change it fairly frequently, with this in mind, from one thing to another. . . . Often indeed medicine must do one thing at one time, and the next moment do the contrary.[2]

The dangers posed by poorly guided cures should not provide an excuse to avoid diets in general—or Grape Cures in particular—but should prompt us to embark on them fully informed. Too many miraculous healings have been obtained for these healing procedures to be abandoned.

This information concerning healing crises appears to be diametrically opposed to what Brandt espoused, insofar as she sometimes recommended following her diet "until the patient has been reduced to a veritable skeleton."

Other authors from the early twentieth century—and even those from earlier eras—have recommended perseverance "to the very end," and their personal experiences seem to justify their assertions. Current wisdom, however, warns against the will to maintain a harsh diet until a cure has been effected. Why is this so?

It could be that this difference does not stem from ignorance about the healing processes, but rather from the vast difference between the physical capacities of modern humans and those of the early twentieth century. There are several levels of meaning here.

In our time, we meet fewer and fewer of those "forces of nature"—individuals of imposing and resistant physique, capable of undergoing any ordeal without incurring much damage. The sedentary habits and overeating that characterize our era have made our bodies lazy and weak, and heavily diminished our resistance. When we must deal with a diet, our scant vital forces are insufficient to perform the tasks of autolysis and elimination imposed by the diet.

On the other hand, modern food is subject to numerous refining processes that often leave it poor in vitamins, trace elements, and other valuable substances. The resulting deficiencies starve the tissues of substances like vitamins that support autolysis by stimulating enzyme activity. Because the body's reserves are reduced, autolysis quickly reaches its limits and stops.

The twenty-first-century human being will rapidly reach phases IV and V, suffering malnutrition and vitality loss, and despite a determination to stick with the diet, will not have the physical resources to do so.

Another point to consider is the degree of chemical pollution to which modern bodies are subjected. Air pollution, water pollution, soil contamination, insecticides, herbicides, pesticides, fungicides, preservatives, food colorings, pharmaceutical medications . . . all contribute to a new kind of poisoning. Many of these are synthetic substances as well, meaning they were artificially created in the laboratory and are unknown to our bodies, which have great difficulty integrating them into our biological circuitry.

Substances like these can actively oppose enzymatic activity and greatly disturb the body's normal biochemical functions, including autolysis. This obstruction property is known as *damming* in homeopathy, and it is joined by yet another form of blocking: a number of chemical pollutants, both metals and other substances, have been found to exert an "anti-vitamin" effect, or a chelation of trace elements. In other words, these substances block and neutralize the activity of vitamins and trace elements. How, under these conditions, can autolysis proceed unhindered?

These obstacles do not make it impossible to follow diets, but they do make diets more difficult to handle. The lack of physical resources mandates a shorter cure duration and thus more repetitions over time. However, beneficial results can be achieved with this approach.

INDICATIONS OF THE CURE

Indications for the Grape Cure flow logically out of its contraindications. Any individual who does not suffer from a metabolic weakness for dealing with acids can take the cure and draw great benefits from it. By interpreting the healing crises correctly, by distinguishing a true crisis from a false one, an individual following the cure can stop at the right time and gain the full benefit.

Trying to pinpoint the type of patient for whom this cure is recommended may be wasted effort. The Grape Cure is not specific; it is not indicated more for one disease than for another; it acts on illnesses of all kinds with purifying and regenerative effects. The questions to ask are whether the individual enjoys grapes and whether that person's body can tolerate them. What has made the Grape Cure so popular is that many people enjoy and will continue to enjoy the flavor of grapes, even during the long weeks of the cure.

7

A Practical Guide to the Cure

To the extent that people can take responsibility for their own health and strive to follow a cure, persevere in their efforts, and surmount the inherent obstacles, they can derive optimum benefits from a cure by educating themselves about it. Unfortunately, too often this does not happen. Many people follow cures, but they follow them *ineffectively*. They are unaware of some details and they leave out other aspects that—if they were included—would enable greater success in the search for healing and well-being.

The practical guide that follows remedies these shortcomings by summarizing the most important points of the cure and demonstrating how it can be most effectively put into practice. The recommendations provided here are not only valid for the Grape Cure, but are transferable to other mono diets as well.

PREPARATION FOR THE CURE

Preparation *must* precede the cure. Over the course of a fast or a mono diet, copious wastes will be extracted from tissues and these will seek an exit from the body. They must find a route to the outside. To effect this, the excretory organs—the body's exits—must be open and functioning correctly. If the intestines are blocked, the liver congested, the kidneys fatigued, and the skin sealed, wastes will be unable to leave. Consequently, they will merely change location inside the body. The internal cellular environment will not be cleansed and healing will not occur. To the contrary, the patient might feel even worse. Opening the excretory organs at the start of a fast or mono diet—even before the start—is critical. A slight reduction of food intake prior to launching the diet also is helpful, preparing the body for the diet. This will be discussed further under Beginning a Restricted Diet, starting on page 90.

Opening the Excretory Organs

Opening the excretory organs simply means freeing them of wastes that burden their tissues and maintaining their proper function by stimulating them to begin work. Brandt talks primarily about the opening of the intestinal tract. To provide a complete picture, we will also discuss opening the liver, kidneys, skin, and lungs.

INTESTINES

The intestinal excretory organ can be opened and kept that way with the use of enemas, colonic irrigations, purges, and gentle plant laxatives.

Enemas

An enema consists of introducing water into the colon, where it dissolves solids and eliminates them with the expelled liquid. An enema kit can be purchased in health stores, pharmacies, and other specialty shops to assist in introducing this liquid. Kits include a half-gallon container for the water, a long rubber tube, and a cannula (tube suitable for insertion into the anus) fitted with a stopcock valve for regulating the flow of liquid.

Bring a half gallon of water to a boil in which you will then steep five chamomile tea bags or a dozen dried flowers. Let this infusion cool until it has reached a temperature of 95–98°F (35–37°C). Remove tea bags and filter any leaves before filling the half-gallon container with the liquid. Place the bag higher than the body so that gravity will provide enough water pressure to help the liquid enter the intestines.

The cannula is introduced into the anus with the stopcock closed. Kneel on all fours and lean head and torso forward and down.

Open the valve and let the water enter the intestines. Breath deeply and slightly alter position—or even massage the abdomen along the path of the colon—to help the liquid penetrate.

If the water pressure in the intestines is too strong or painful, close the valve for a minute or two.

Once the water has been introduced, the cannula is removed. The liquid should be retained for several minutes to allow the stools to liquefy. Then evacuate the intestinal contents. This is generally achieved in several waves.

Half-gallon enemas can be performed on a daily basis during a fast or mono diet, per Brandt's suggestion, or twice a week over a period of two to three weeks. After several enemas have been administered, they can be replaced by ingestion of plant laxatives (see Gentle Laxatives section on page 88). During the mono diet, neither enemas nor laxatives should be employed if the food chosen for the diet is sufficiently laxative.

Colonic Irrigations

A colonic irrigation is similar to an enema, the difference being that the cannula contains two conduits, one allowing liquid to flow in and the other for it to leave without delay. Liquid is first introduced and held until it fills the entire colon. Then a valve on the outgoing tube is opened to permit evacuation of the fluid and materials from the colon while continuing to introduce additional water through the in-valve. This creates a current that constantly renews the fluid base for evacuation and also sets up a slight current that has a scouring effect on wastes affixed to the intestinal walls.

Colonic irrigations are a highly effective method for cleansing the colon, but they are not to be done at home; they require specialized equipment and the supervision of a medical practitioner.

Purging

Before initiating enemas, a purge is recommended to free the intestines of the bulk of their waste. Many purging formulas are available, with a number of commercial variations sold ready to use. As the procedure is physically rigorous, it is recommended only for people with strong intestines and it should be employed only at the start of the cure. For people with sensitive intestines, it is better to use gentle laxatives. (Those with sensitive intestines will generally be aware of the fact because they will have pains immediately after eating certain foods, such as spicy meals and too many fruits.)

Dr. Ed. Bertholet, of Lausanne, Switzerland, who was famous for his book on fasting *(Le retour à la santé par le jeûne)* recommended the following purgative formula: Blend 40–55 grams of magnesium citrate and 10–15 grams of sodium citrate in approximately 1 pint of lukewarm water. Drink within a half an hour. The effect will be felt within several hours.

Gentle Laxatives

A variety of medicinal plants can gently stimulate intestinal function and encourage them to empty. As these substances are neither irritating nor rigorous for the intestines, they can be used daily during the cure. As noted previously, they may replace enemas.

Alder buckthorn: Alder buckthorn is an excellent plant laxative whose gentle action allows even pregnant women to use it, on the advice of their physician. Because of its unpleasant taste, it is preferable to take it in drops in the form of a tincture (rather than as an infusion or decoction): Take 30–50 drops of buckthorn tincture with water just before bedtime. The laxative will take effect by the next morning. Alternatively, take 15–30 drops three times a day with water before meals.

Castor oil: Castor oil can be a laxative or a purgative, depending on the dose. Whereas many laxatives act primarily on the colon, castor oil acts on the small intestine. The disagreeable taste is no longer an obstacle; castor oil can now be purchased in capsules of varying dosage.

LIVER

The liver filters wastes out of the blood, and neutralizes and destroys toxins, poisons, germs, and diseased cells as well. The liver is stimulated primarily with medicinal plants.

Dandelion: For a tincture, take 10–50 drops with water three times a day before meals. In tablet form, take 1–3 tablets with water, three times a day before meals. As a decoction, steep a large handful of leaves and roots in a half gallon of water; boil for two minutes, then steep for ten minutes; drink several cups a day.

Boldo: The leaves of this Chilean tree are effective for draining the liver. Create an infusion by mixing 1 teaspoon of

Boldo per cup of water and steep ten minutes. For a tincture, take 20–50 drops with water three times a day before meals.

KIDNEYS

Drinking more water than usual (more than 2 liters a day) and ingesting plants that stimulate diuresis will help to increase the elimination of toxins by the kidneys. Thanks to the diuretic action of plants such as pilosella and the leaves of birch and ash trees, urine is excreted more often and in larger volume. The urine's color also gets darker, because of the amount of toxins it carries.

Pilosella: An excellent diuretic. Take 30–50 drops of pilosella tincture in a little water three times a day before meals.

Birch or ash leaves: Make an infusion with 1 handful of leaves for $1/2$ gallon of water; steep ten minutes and drink as desired.

SKIN

The skin will open more easily with the help of saunas and hot baths. Linden, borage, elderberry leaves, chamomile, and wild pansies, isolated or in herb-tea blends, encourage the skin to eliminate wastes and toxins. Create an infusion with 2–3 teaspoons of an herb in 1 cup of water; steep for ten minutes.

LUNGS

An increase in the elimination of mucus, phlegm, and other waste products by the respiratory tract can be obtained with plants like thyme and plantain. By liquefying these colloidal wastes, these plants make them easier to be expectorated, or coughed, out of the body.

Thyme: Make an infusion with 1 pinch of thyme per cup of water; steep for ten minutes; drink three cups a day.

Plantain: Create an infusion with 1–2 teaspoons per cup of water; steep ten minutes; drink three cups a day.

Beginning a Restricted Diet

As newly opened excretory organs (by virtue of the plants previously discussed) act on circulating wastes that are easy to eliminate, and mono diets and fasts will work on deeply embedded wastes, a strict diet is not called for during the preparation stage. Much of the work of eliminating toxins will be performed by the action of draining before the patient begins the actual cure.

Some small dietary restrictions have their uses, however, given that they can prepare the body for future dietary restrictions, reduce the shock of changing the diet, and accustom the body to functioning on reduced intake.

These preparatory restrictions include principally stimulants (coffee, tobacco, alcohol), meat, and cooked dishes. The preparatory reduced diet will consist primarily of raw and cooked vegetables, grains, and dairy products. This light but complete diet will be followed throughout the preparation stage, which can extend for several weeks if there is no urgency to begin the cure sooner. Brandt suggested a rapid entry into the diet with a fast included in the preparation stage, but she directed her advice to gravely ill patients for whom all speed was necessary.

THE CURE ITSELF

The Practice of the Fast

Although Brandt lists fasting under preparation for the cure, because it is such an integral part of the Grape Cure or any other mono diet, it is placed here as a main element of the cure.

As we have seen, by ingesting no nutrients during the fast,

the body will find nourishment in its own tissues. Only water and unsweetened herb teas are allowed. Liquids ingested this way are not nutritious and serve only as the essential replacements for the fluids that are used up and eliminated. Herb teas retain their vitalizing and purifying properties, but do not contribute nutritionally.

Water—a good spring or mineral water—as well as herb teas can be drunk as desired, depending on the faster's thirst. Be certain, however, that enough liquid is consumed to encourage the transport and elimination of toxins. Drink a minimum of three liters a day. Drinks can be ingested hot, which may be advisable to help a faster maintain body heat (in cases of cold sensitivity). This intake of calories "free of charge" (meaning the body does not need to produce them from food) is a welcome energy benefit.

KEEPING THE EXCRETORY
ORGANS OPEN DURING THE CURE
To ensure the constant elimination of toxins released by autolysis, the subject must ensure that excretory organs remain open through the duration of the fast and mono diet.

This is accomplished by the same means as those employed in the preparation stage. Use purifying plants and enemas (but not purges) regularly, based on needs.

STIMULATING THE METABOLISM
Remaining prone, in bed or on a sofa, during a fast or mono diet is not necessary. To the contrary, avoiding "external movement" brings on an equivalent slowdown in "internal movement." Organ functions, blood circulation, and cellular exchanges are improved by physical activity. Here, too, this activity must be adapted to the individual's strength and needs.

We should keep in mind, however, that organ function does tend to slow down during a fast, given that organs are no longer stimulated by food intake. Engaging in moderate physical activity is, therefore, all the more important, as are light hydrotherapy, massage with a brush or loofah, deep breathing, and so on.

WHEN HEALING CRISES OCCUR

We have learned that these crises are natural. When they occur, support the excretory organ involved by encouraging its work with medicinal plants and activities that stimulate it to drain. Take a session in the sauna to induce heavy sweating, or soak in a hot bath to open the skin; drink infusions made from plants with expectorant properties to free respiratory passages; drink quantities of fluid to flush the kidneys and reduce the concentration of urine; use an enema to further empty the intestines.

If the crisis is too painful, it is also possible to divert wastes toward another excretory organ. To do this, stimulate one of the eliminatory organs that has not been overwhelmed by the crisis, and keep that alternate organ fully open to draw toxins to it. This can be done by employing the opening methods discussed in the preparation phase of the regimen. For example, wastes of the skin can be diverted to the kidneys and vice versa. The lungs are relieved by detouring toxins toward the liver and intestines. If the healing crisis is long and too arduous, verify that the faster has not reached the malnutrition stage by resuming slight food intake and observing how the crisis responds.

Urgent Signs to Stop Fasting

In addition to the return of authentic hunger, the following signs are indications that a fast should be interrupted:
- The breath has an acetone odor (like apples or ether). This signifies that the body is no longer breaking down fats and is threatened by an acetone crisis. You should quickly begin to eat sweet foods.
- Sudden, substantial weight loss, accompanied by a loss of vitality.
- Total, persistent depression.
- Total, persistent exhaustion.
- Insomnia or nightmares, night after night.

The Mono Diet in Practice
CHOOSING THE FOOD

Given that a mono diet can last for weeks, the food it is based on must be chosen with care. Several criteria should be considered: the beneficial properties of the food itself; its availability during the season when the cure is used; and, most importantly, the preference of the person following the cure.

As we have seen, the grape is an excellent food for mono diets because it is a pleasure to eat, and it possesses valuable nutritive substances and important healing properties. Other foods can be used; these are among the most beneficial.

- Vegetables: artichokes, beets, cabbage, carrots, celery, fennel, lettuce, potatoes, pumpkin, turnips
- Fruits: apples, apricots, bananas, cherries, melons, peaches, pears, strawberries, watermelon

- Dried fruits: dates, figs, raisins
- Nuts: almonds, hazelnuts
- Grains: barley, corn, rice
- Light dairy products: curdled milk, whey

Fruits and vegetables can be consumed raw, cooked, or as juice. Grains are always consumed cooked, with slight salt permitted. People who metabolize acids poorly should not choose fresh fruits or tomatoes.

It is extremely important that the foods are ripe, untreated, and organically grown. Foods contraindicated for these diets are meat, fish, eggs, beans, and sweets.

QUANTITIES

The selected food is to be eaten at every meal. It is preferable to eat at the accustomed mealtimes, as the stomach will expect nourishment at these times. Small snacks—always of the same food—can be eaten as needed.

Food should be eaten until hunger is satisfied, taking care not to overeat. There is little chance of extreme overindulgence, though, as eating only one food causes the body to feel quickly satiated. Obviously, dates or almonds will be eaten in smaller quantities than grapes, given the richness of these fruits and nuts.

IN THE EVENT OF APPETITE LOSS

When the food becomes boring, the person following the mono diet can wait for appetite to return or try cooking the food if it has been consumed raw, or vice versa. Another food in the same category (replacing a fruit with a fruit, a vegetable with a vegetable) can also be substituted. The value of the diet will be somewhat less because the digestive tract will have more work to do adapting to the change in food, but it will permit the person following the cure to remain on the diet and will still elicit a good result.

In fact, some mono diets change the food each day, some at every meal. Understanding the principles of the restriction imposed by a mono diet is critical. It can then be adapted to the particularities of the person who is following the cure.

LENGTH OF THE MONO DIET

The length of a mono diet is based on its therapeutic purpose and the person's physical capacities, willpower, and so on. There is no fixed duration. Each diet must be adapted on a case-by-case basis, and most often the duration will be determined over the course of the cure itself.

COMING OFF THE CURE

Resumption of a Regular Diet

Ending a cure correctly by gradually introducing the standard diet is important. The digestive tract cannot be called on suddenly to resume normal activity after a long period of repose. A transitional period must be provided so it can gradually recover a working rhythm. The length of this transition will be proportionate to the length of the cure: a transition of two or three meals works for a cure of several days, but two to three days are needed to transition out of a cure that lasted several weeks.

The resumption of a regular diet starts with light and easily digested foods (fruits, vegetables, soups, gruels, potatoes). Later, dairy products, meats, and eggs can be reintroduced. If foods like meat or a cooked meal are eaten as soon as the cure ends, indigestion will result. The digestive mucous membranes will become irritated and inflamed by insufficiently digested foods. The individual coming off the cure will need nutrition but be unable to eat because he or she feels ill.

The Gradual Halt of Drainers

When resuming a regular diet, drainers should not be stopped suddenly. The body has become accustomed to functioning with their help during the cure, and now needs time to get used to functioning without their aid. It will do so, but it needs time to adapt gradually. The plant doses recommended should be reduced slowly and the frequency with which they are taken can be spaced out over the course of two or three days, depending on the length of the cure that preceded it. The excretory organs will be revitalized and fortified by draining during the cure.

Practical Guide Summary

Preparation for the Cure

Opening the excretory organs

- Intestines: enemas, colonic irrigation, purges, or gentle laxatives
- Liver: hepatic medicinal plants
- Kidneys: diuretic medicinal plants and drinking large amounts of fluid
- Skin: sauna or hot baths, sweat-inducing medicinal plants
- Lungs: expectorant-acting medicinal plants

Beginning a restricted diet

- Reduce intake of caffeine, tobacco, alcohol, meat, and cooked dishes

The Cure Itself

The fast and the mono diet

- Keep the excretory organs open
- Stimulate the metabolism with physical exercise, oxygenation, and light hydrotherapy

Coming off the Cure

- Gradually and gently reintroduce food
- Gradually stop the use of drainers

Part Two

THE GRAPE CURE

By Johanna Brandt

Note: In 1928 Johanna Brandt wrote *The Grape Cure* based on the discoveries she had made experimenting on her body in search of a cure for the stomach cancer from which she suffered. Her book is reproduced here, reformatted and abridged. Her text was re-sequenced to increase understanding of the material. Where it was necessary, clarifying information has been added to make the information as accessible as possible. There is much to be learned from the remarkable healings that have resulted from this cure; however, Brandt was not a doctor and many advances have been made in the field of medicine since the 1920s. As with any remedy, it is advisable to consult a qualified health care professional before beginning treatment. —C.V.

Preface

You are not on a Grape Cure when you are eating other foods at the same time. The Grape Cure is the exclusive ingestion of these fruits. No one expects you to live on grapes for the rest of your life. When the grape has done its work, you can go back to your normal habits, but make sure that they are not abnormal. You do not change your religion when you go on the Grape Cure; it's simply a change of diet.

No one tries to give a drowning person a swimming lesson. Study the Grape Cure while you are well. Be prepared.

JOHANNA BRANDT

In the present desperate need of the world, I am offering this book as my contribution toward the solution of the cancer problem. It is founded on personal experience and is put forward more as a prevention of cancer than as a cure.

On the eve of the grape season, the time is propitious for verifying what I claim in these pages—to wit, that the grape is a natural remedy to cancer, tuberculosis, and other diseases. It would be wrong to give false hope to the sick. It is not enough to eat grapes to cure cancer, you must do more than that. The toxins stirred up by the chemical activity of the grape should be eliminated and this can be done by applying the natural treatment methods I have tried to explain in these pages.

It is my duty to stress the fact that among those who have reached the final stages of this terrible disease, very few have a chance of being healed. Their condition will improve, their suffering will be relieved to some extent, but there is not enough time for the grape to purify their blood, the essential condition for stopping the course of the disease.

Under favorable circumstances, advanced cases of cancer have been pronounced cured by these means. But when patients come to us in a desperate condition, after having undergone several operations, and what remains is skin and bones, the Grape Cure and treatments by natural methods can no longer save them.

I am not giving instructions for the treatment of advanced cases; I cannot assume more responsibility for those sufferers who treat themselves, but I seriously recommend the reader to carefully study the following information.

A large part of this information is based on my personal experience, but I have also drawn from reputable sources in the domain of medicine-free healing, in both England and America, and in fact all over the world. I have a debt of gratitude to all the inspired authors of valuable works, a debt that can never be repaid. The list of their names would be too long to be published here.

8
The Fourth of July 1927

It was midwinter when I left my home in the Transvaal to bring the message of the discovery of a remedy for cancer to the United States of America.

Nothing could have been more dreary than that dusty little platform of our provincial town. Something clutched my heart when I looked on the wan faces of the children who had helped to get Mother ready for her strange expedition. When would I see them again? Matters were not improved by the fact that my husband's face was missing. He was away from home on affairs connected with our church.

It was the 4th of July—the American Day of Independence. This was a mere coincidence. The date had not been prearranged because of its significance but because it fitted in with the lectures I had to deliver in Bloemfontein and Cape Town before sailing for England by the *Windsor Castle*.

It was a good omen, I told the children. America was a free country politically, and an independent, powerful, progressive, rich, and enlightened nation. But it was not free from disease. I had no doubt whatsoever that this free nation would accept my message, and, accepting it, be blessed with a new emancipation—a wonderful deliverance from disease and premature death. I tried to conjure up visions of the blessed and beautiful state of the world when, through America, a perishing humanity had been saved from suffering and the poverty that so often follows the wake of disease.

In Cape Town, after one of my lectures, an astrologer who happened to be present volunteered the information that the planetary influences were against my enterprise. I was earnestly advised to cancel my voyage and return to the Transvaal.

This was discouraging! To hide my depression, I smiled and said:

"I shall overcome all planetary and other evil influences, by the grace of God!"

The tranquil majesty of Table Mountain enveloped me in a parting benediction.

Disappointment followed my wake. Every plan was frustrated; my funds ran low and I was so much delayed in England and Europe that it was the end of November before I arrived in New York.

Perhaps some day the story may be written of how in the end, by the grace of God, every obstacle was overcome.

The first three months in America were difficult indeed. I found to my great disappointment that the Medical Practice Act of the State of New York was tyrannical in the extreme. Much time was lost in constructing a plan by which I could demonstrate the efficacy of the Grape Cure.

As a law-abiding citizen of South Africa, I had no desire to come into conflict with the law of a strange land. There was nothing to do, therefore, but to secure the cooperation of registered medical men and carry out my healing campaign under their protection.

But would it be possible to find medical men who would be willing to supervise test cases under an unknown system of healing?

The time spent in searching for them was not lost. I visited many people and institutions, presented letters of introduction, delivered private lectures, and worked up many valuable connections. My main activity, however, was writing. The little portable Corona typewriter that accompanied me everywhere since 1916 was nearly worn out with letters I wrote to the editors of leading newspapers and magazines, the heads of healing movements, the pastors of churches and—last but not least—the most prominent medical men connected with the campaign against cancer.

But these efforts met with no success. The months went by and I did not get even an acknowledgment of the receipt of any of my communications.

Two years before, when I was lecturing in Cape Town, I met a fine American woman who was interested in healing and who still had time, on her trip around the world, to help me with my work. We became close friends. Her home in Long Island received me after I landed in New York.

"It is God who built the nest of the blind bird."

I still have the latchkey of that home. The refuge is always ready.

Those who have drunk deeply of the cup of homesickness will understand. But this was no ordinary homesickness. It was not longing for home and loved ones, or a yearning for the "slumbering, sunlit vastness" of South Africa. It was a state of mental and spiritual anguish charged with unfathomable suffering of all the ages. It was my utter helplessness.

To hold the key to the solution of most of the problems of life and to have it rejected, untried, as worthless—that is to pass through the dark night of the soul. To have a mockery of worldly splendors thrust upon one as a substitute for an ideal—that is the temptation in the wilderness. To offer the gift of deliverance from pain, freely, without money, and without price and to see it spurned—that is crucifixion—Calvary.

THE TURNING OF THE TIDE

Among others, I had a letter of introduction to the father of naturopathy in America, Dr. Benedict Lust, and when I placed my difficulties before him he advised me to approach Mr. Bernarr Macfadden, editor of the *Evening Graphic* and the famous magazine *Physical Culture*.

Mr. Macfadden received me very kindly. In spite of the fact that I was still withholding the secret of the Grape Cure (until it could be brought forward in such a way that it could never be disputed), he listened attentively to my story and finally invited me to write an account of the discovery for the *Evening Graphic*.

What seemed to impress him most was the fact that I was prepared to undergo an exploratory operation to prove my claim, for I have always maintained that the scars of the malignant growth were still present in my body.

This proof of my sincerity touched him and he made a special feature of my case in a full-page article in the *Evening Graphic* of January 21, 1928.

9

The Story of the Discovery

In the Magazine Section of the New York *Evening Graphic* on January 21, 1928, my article was published as follows:

> I was born in the heart of South Africa in 1876. Over fifty years ago, my forefathers were heavy meat eaters and practically lived on game, as did most South Africans in those days. I do not know whether this has anything to do with the fact that cancer is the greatest scourge of our country, but I think so.
>
> There was a lot of cancer in my father's family and my mother died of cancer in 1916. The doctors tell us that the disease is not hereditary. This may be true, but the predisposing causes of cancer in my mother's body may have been present in my own.
>
> It is not unreasonable to assume this. Be that as it may, as long as I can remember I suffered from gastric trouble, bilious attacks, and stomach ulcers.
>
> It is cruel, when one is of a highly romantic temperament, to have to turn one's internal organs inside out for public inspection.

Why could it not have been something less prosaic? Heart disease, lung trouble, or a delicate throat? But stomach! A reeking, fermenting stomach, and a blatantly conspicuous one at that!

After the anguishing spectacle of my mother's martyrdom, I had one shock after another. Life became a ghastly nightmare, and through it all I was conscious of a gnawing pain at the left side of my stomach.

Cancer? I was not afraid of it. In my ignorance, I thought I had reached the limit of human endurance. I saw in cancer a possible release.

A friend, meeting my husband one day, inquired after my health, and was so much struck by his reply that she repeated it to me: "What must I say about my wife? The hope of death is keeping her alive, and the fear of life is nearly killing her."

The hope of death! That was it. But I was puzzled to know how my secret had been discovered.

My plan of action was carefully prearranged. I would allow nothing to be done that could prolong life. If it were really cancer, no medicines would be taken to check the disease. No injections. No drugs to alleviate pain. And, under no circumstances, the application of the surgeon's knife.

At this time, a little book was put into my hands, *The Fasting Cure,* by Upton Sinclair. It thrilled me. A new hope surged through me, the hope of relief from suffering. Here was something that appealed to my common sense. Something constructive—Nature Cure.

The book set the fasting ball rolling in our house. I fasted for seven days. The result was disappointing.

STARTED FASTING CLASS

Undaunted, I fasted again and persuaded everyone else to fast. In time, I set up a fasting business, free of charge. Any one and every one could fast for nothing under my supervision. I became highly experienced and seemed to cure every one, except myself.

The study of one system of healing led to another. Our home was stacked with the best American books and magazines on the science of spinal adjustment, German water cures, Swiss sun bathing, Russian fruit cures, and Oriental works on the science of deep breathing.

A flame had been lighted that nothing could extinguish. It was a pleasure to see our large family of sons and daughters growing tall, strong, and athletic. I once overheard the following fragment of a good-humored argument between two small sons:

"You talk more nonsense in a day than Charlie Chaplin does in a week. Eat more fruit, man! You will feel much better."

"Fruit! What you want is a jolly good fast."

We chewed raw carrots and peanuts until our jaws ached. We began the day with spinal exercises and finished it by sleeping outside.

The whole family joined hands with me in the campaign against disease. Our fortune was spent in building up a system of natural healing so perfect in its simplicity and economy that it would meet the needs of the farming population in the remotest regions of South Africa.

I wrote books and answered thousands of letters, but under it all I knew that my own internal trouble was not responding to Nature Cure.

NINE YEAR BATTLE FOR LIFE

My battle for life lasted nine years. I fasted myself to a skeleton. I fasted beyond the starvation point, which is a most unusual proceeding, consuming my own live tissues in the effort to destroy the growth. With every fast, the growth was unmistakably checked. But it was not destroyed. On the contrary, it seemed to take a new hold on me whenever I broke the fast.

Because I took the wrong foods.

HOW CANCER THRIVES

I knew exactly what was taking place. I knew that it was wrong to undermine the system by injurious fasting and then to nourish the growth by wrong feeding.

What was I to do? There was no one to advise me, but while experimenting on myself, I was learning something new every day.

Among other things, I learned that cancer thrives on every form of animal food—the more impure, the better. I suffered from horrible and disgusting cravings for blood—for beef and pork and rich blood-sausages—for stimulating and highly seasoned foods.

The growth was now pushing its way through the diaphragm, toward the heart and left lung. I seemed to see it like a red octopus feeding on the impure blood at the base of the lung. Breathing became difficult. I spat blood occasionally.

One night in August, 1920, I had a terrible attack of vomiting and purging, with excruciating pain. Toward morning, I brought up a quantity of half-digested blood.

IN SERIOUS CONDITION

Matters were becoming serious, and the thought of the death certificate and possible complications troubled me. I sent for our family physician.

He ordered me to lie still in bed for three months. Under his supervision, I fasted twelve days. Plenty of time now to write glowing accounts of the wonders of Nature Cure to distant correspondents.

More than ever, I realized the importance of saving my own life in order to convince and try to save others.

It was under this fast that I first noticed an ominous sign, the presence of digested blood—known in medical circles as "coffee grounds"—in the stools after the use of the enema. Still more disconcerting to find that I no longer put on weight on breaking the fast.

Toward the end of 1920, I seemed to be fasting chronically, four, seven, ten days, and finally three weeks in December.

Nothing has been said in this article about the mental aspect of healing. The subject is too big. It forms the most thrilling story of my life, but I must be now content to state that I became super-conscious. I had unerring "hunches" and cultivated a bowing acquaintance with my subliminal self—whatever that may be.

All this fasting brought about a slight improvement and I dragged through 1921 somehow. Then in November, I was persuaded by my doctor to go into the General Hospital in Johannesburg for an x-ray examination.

Many plates were taken, and a noted surgeon pronounced his verdict—the stomach was being divided in two by a vicious, fibrous growth. An immediate operation was recommended as the only means of prolonging my life. This I refused.

The famous doctor who was operating in the x-ray department was much interested in my experiences and invited me to his house for another x-ray examination if I found myself still in the land of the living after six months.

Encouraged by the mark of sympathy, I fasted three weeks in December, drinking pure water only and lying in the morning sun. When, after six months, I went under the x-ray again, no trace of the growth could be found!

BUT PAIN REMAINED

I assured the doctor, however, that the pain was still there and told him that I was looking for a food that would answer a threefold purpose, i.e.: destroy the growth effectually, eliminate the poison, and build new tissue.

The three years that followed were years of great suffering, but I kept on fasting and dieting alternately, and in 1925, after a seven-day fast, I accidentally discovered a food that had the miraculous effect of healing me completely within six weeks.

The publication of this discovery will be of more value after the particulars set forth in this article have been proved to be facts.

I therefore call upon the medical council to have an exploratory operation performed. The gravity of the disease can only be estimated by an examination of the extent of the damage done, and then only can the efficacy of the cure be established.

A method that may cure cancer may cure almost any other disease. What is more, it may prevent cancer and almost every other disease.

While I was experimenting on myself, I was often discouraged by the thought that very few people would be able to undergo such rigorous treatment.

But it is the sum total of my experience that I hope to bring before the public. Fasting for such a long period was unnecessary. The mistakes I made need not be made by other patients. Our system of healing has been greatly modified by the discovery of the food cure. And while the patient is undergoing the cure for his or her own particular complaint, nature is secretly restoring and rejuvenating every part of the body.

The senses become abnormally acute; dim eyes brighten; faded hair takes on new gloss; the lifeless, hopeless voice becomes vibrant, magnetic; and the complexion clears.

I have seen beautiful sets of teeth, loose in their suppuration sockets, become steady and fixed within a few weeks, the gums free of pyorrhea within a few months.

I have watched our old people getting young and our young people becoming superbly beautiful, and with every new entrancing revelation of the wonders of Nature Cure I have dedicated my life anew to this joyous work of spreading the good news.

The above article created widespread interest. An afflicted nation stirred to the chord of hope that had been struck. I was overwhelmed with correspondence and visits.

This led to unexpected developments.

That Saturday morning was a landmark. I had an informal luncheon party in my hotel to celebrate the publication of an article that I believed would revolutionize healing throughout the world. It was amusing to listen to the outcry of my friends against the proposed operation. It had gone out in the form of a challenge to the medical fraternity and, if they accepted it, I would be bound in honor to submit to it.

On the 21st day of January, a stranger called at my hotel—a medical man and a surgeon! The *Evening Graphic* was only a few hours old and already a prospective executioner had arrived on the scene.

But this kindly, enthusiastic man had no designs upon me. The purpose of his visit was to encourage me, to urge me to be steadfast, not to be dissuaded from my plan. Nothing could be finer than such evidence of devotion to a cause, he said.

Afterward I found out that he was a member of the medical profession of exceptionally high standing, and when letters came pouring in from every part of the United States and Canada, in response to my article, I consulted him.

From other medical men, there was no response to my challenge. One month I waited and then, as no surgeon had volunteered to examine my claims, I formally withdrew my challenge.

Another and better way had in the meantime been found of demonstrating the efficacy of my discovery. If others afflicted with cancer could be cured, then my theory would be proven.

The many heartbreaking appeals for relief could not be ignored. As the laws of the land did not forbid me to tell the story of how I cured myself, I simply related my experiences and described the procedure I had adopted. People treated by my methods recovered. They in their turn told their relatives and friends—always with the same results.

Correspondents clamored for information about the "Grape Cure." At first we sent out typed copies, but when the demand became excessive, we had a four-page leaflet prepared. Five editions of this were printed. Newspapers in distant states reproduced it and inquiries came pouring in thick and fast. This leaflet, which was distributed free of charge, became famous.

When it became necessary to have a secretary, a woman with great executive ability stepped forward and offered her services. Her rooms were placed at my disposal for the reception of visitors. Our surprise may be imagined when we found that the physician, who had called at my hotel, had his office in the same building.

The cancer patients who came to us were referred to him.

Other doctors appeared to try the cure on their cancer patients. These experimental treatments were given for free.

10

Directions for the Grape Cure

FIRST STAGE: IMPORTANT
PREPARATION FOR THE CURE

Fasting means only drinking water. Enemas help to quickly eliminate harmful substances from the body. This way you can avoid hunger and mainly prevent the released toxins from being absorbed into the circulation.

Don't eat foods that are difficult to digest before beginning preparations for the cure. To prepare the system for the change of diet, fast for two or three days, drinking plenty of pure water and taking a daily enema of lukewarm water. This preparation is essential.

This fast can avoid complications, for the stomach is cleared of poisons and fermentation. In this way grapes can begin their work more quickly. This fast is even more necessary if the patient has been taking a lot of medicines. It is better to abstain from taking any medication during the cure if considered safe to do so by a qualified health care professional.

When going on any detoxification cure for any illness, you will experience elimination crises. These can cause headaches, nausea, diarrhea, and the illness itself seems to get worse. It is recommended that you get a lot of rest during the first days.

If the patient is unaccustomed to enemas or is too ill to do them, he can ask for the help of a nurse or other third party. Half-gallon containers can be found at the pharmacy or drugstore, where you can also learn how to use enemas.

No exceptions should be made when fasting because even a morsel of sugar can cause the gastric juices to start working and cause hunger pangs and fermentation.

If someone says that she cannot tolerate the fast or the grapes, it means she does not understand the reactions, or she started the Grape Cure without taking the necessary preparation.

Enemas

You have to learn how to use enemas correctly. Ingesting water through the rectum is almost as natural as it is through the mouth, provided neither salt nor soap is used. The use of enemas will not paralyze the rectum or the intestines like artificial purgatives can do.

Fasting

The best natural medicine is the fast. Because this subject requires some study, I can give only a brief overview of its principles.

Fasting means purifying the blood, which causes the germs of illness and death to perish. These germs cannot survive in pure blood, because they live on impurities.

A sensible fast is not synonymous with agonizing privation.

For the patient, this is a change of diet. The vital organs are nourished by the blood, by the supplies Mother Nature holds in reserve for such circumstances, more specifically the fat layers collected between the internal organs and beneath the skin. These reserves are used to maintain the functions of the heart, the brain, the lungs, and other organs while toxins are eliminated. A fasting cure, practiced scientifically, magnificently activates the excretory organs.

The Quickest Relief

I used to think that fasting was the quickest relief we knew. But how much I have learned since 1921! There is no comparison between the fasting method and the Grape Cure. I believe that nothing can take the place of the complete fast in acute disease, but the fast only partially eliminates the inorganic deposits by which chronic diseases are often caused. Perhaps that is the reason why we cannot be cured by fasting only. So fast, but finish the process by the purification offered by the Grape Cure.

SECOND STAGE: THE EXCLUSIVE GRAPE DIET

Finally the real Grape Cure begins. You will be amazed to see how the wastes of the intestines are still abundant and often black. A large portion of this has been surely glued in the folds of the intestines for years.

The First Grape Meal

After the fast the patient drinks one or two glasses of pure, cold water the first thing in the morning. Half an hour after drinking water, the patient has his first meal of grapes. Wash them well, even leaving them under running water if the grapes have been treated, or let them sit in the water for several hours, then wash them with fresh water. Chew the skins and seeds, if possible, thoroughly and swallow a few of them as food and roughage. (See Why Eat the Skins? for further guidance.)

Timetable

Starting at 8 AM and having a grape meal every two hours till 8 PM would give seven meals daily. This is kept up for a week or two, even a month or two in chronic cases of long standing.* Not longer under any circumstances.

Why Eat the Skins?

The skins—not only of grapes, but of many other fruits, such as apples and pears—contain immensely valuable elements. To throw away the peels would be to deprive the system of the very substances required to build a new and healthy body.

But the skins also form the bulk and roughage that are needed to promote the peristaltic action of the stomach and bowels.

Until the system has learned to utilize the grape, it is advisable to be careful with the seeds and hulls. A normal digestion suffers no inconvenience when the whole grape is used; on the contrary, it is benefited by the valuable properties contained in the seeds and skins apart from the bulk and roughage they provide. But if you have been in the habit of discarding them, they may at first accumulate in the digestive tract and cause constipation. I therefore advise all who are experimenting with the Grape Cure for the first time to begin with the juice and pulp; later add a few of the skins. Chew the skins well in order to extract their essences, but swallow only

---

*[Any chronic illness will take a long time to cure because the illness itself has been in the body for an extensive period of time. Cures lasting longer than a month should be taken only under the supervision of an experienced practitioner. —C.V.]

a few until you are sure that your digestion is able to take care of them. The same applies to the seeds.

When a patient knows that he is suffering from a stomach or intestinal ulcer, he should not swallow grape seeds or skins.

In all cases, use the enema if Nature fails to do her work.

Do not depend on faith for this. The development of faith takes time and there is no time to lose—if it really is a cancer. Throw out the vile poisons. Employ every material means of ridding the system of its gross impurities and you will be surprised to find that in doing this you are developing the more spiritual powers of mind and soul.

Obedience to the dictates of common sense—harmony— has its own rewards.

Bowel Movements

Distressing symptoms occur during the Grape Cure, through the poisons that have been stirred up by the actions of the grape and thrown into the bloodstream. These symptoms may be aggravated in cases in which there is poor elimination. Sufficient stress cannot be laid upon keeping the bowels free by using enemas up to two or three times a day, if necessary.

Many patients complain of becoming constipated under the grape diet; they should not eat the skins of their grapes.

As using laxatives is generally not advised, one can swallow a spoonful of olive oil just before eating grapes. In extreme cases a little olive oil can be introduced into the rectum with a cannula. Some laxatives are not strictly contraindicated as long as they are plant based.

The Enema

It is my belief that the body of the cancer patient contains the most virulent poison, and cancer is the death and disintegration of a given part of a living body.

Under the grape diet, that decomposition is arrested—checked. But the danger is by no means over. The poisons have now been thrown into the bloodstream and carried to every part of the body. Everything must be done to expel them and expel them quickly.

Since the alimentary canal is the main avenue of excretion, the bowels must be attended to first. We recommend the daily use of the enema *unless the grapes act as a laxative.* In some cases they cause constipation until the system has learned to use the skins of the grapes as roughage. Such patients should take an enema of one quart of lukewarm water once or even twice a day, until there is a natural movement of the bowels.

Variety

Any good variety of grapes may be used effectively—purple, green, white, or blue. Hothouse grapes are better than none, and the seedless varieties are excellent. The monotony of the diet may be varied by using many varieties. As they contain distinct elements, it is recommended to eat as many kinds of grape as you can find. Some prefer sour grapes while others like sweet.

The best time for the cure is when the grape season is at its height. If—when you are reading this book—the grape season is at its height, make it a memorable one by converting it into a Festival of Grapes. Perhaps your effort will contribute to a vast movement of regeneration by the Grape Cure, made universal thanks to the many translations that will make it accessible to everyone.

Grape Juice and Raisins

It seems too good to be true, but it is a fact that something has at last been found that effectively solves the problem of what to do when fresh grapes are not procurable.

We have been experimenting with unsweetened, unfermented bottled grape juice and concentrated grape juice to take the place of whole grapes during the winter months. So far, the results have been most gratifying.

Even during the period when whole grapes are abundant, there are times when the patient becomes tired of grapes; frequently also he is too weak to chew them. It therefore gave me double satisfaction to learn that grape juice may take the place of whole grapes.

In critical cases, the patient should fast on water only for a few days or a week or two, using the enema daily as recommended, and then he should live exclusively on grape juice for another short period.

A glassful (one-half pint) is usually given at a meal but more may be taken, if the patient desires.

It has been found that the patient can get along almost as well on grape juice alone as on whole grapes, although whole grapes are preferable when they can be procured. The stomach is accustomed to bulk and is more likely to feel the pangs of hunger when only juice is taken.

As a pleasant variety, raisins (dried grapes) can also be eaten for a while, as something solid to chew. For example, one can drink a glass of grape juice on rising; two hours later, eat a cup or more of raisins; and continue like that at two-hour intervals for the rest of the day. *Do not eat raisins at the same meal you drink juice.* Raisins can be eaten as is or soaked for several hours in cold water; you can eat the raisins and drink the soaking water at one meal (you can use any kind of unsulfured raisin). In cases where it was impossible to procure fresh grapes or grape juice, patients have taken only raisins and drunk this soaking water.

Raisins and fresh grapes need to be taken at two-hour

intervals. If the raisins that have been soaked in water are too sweet, a little lemon juice can be added.

An analysis of grape juice shows that the grape loses none of its healing properties during the process of double sterilization at 194°F (90°C). Health food stores have a number of good brands of unsweetened, unadulterated grape juice.

Quantity

This varies according to the condition, digestion, and occupation of the patient. It is well to begin with a small quantity of one, two, or three ounces of grapes per meal, gradually increasing this to double the amount. In time, about half a pound can be taken at a meal. To make this point quite clear, a minimum of one pound should be used daily and the maximum should not exceed four pounds. Patients taking larger quantities at a meal should allow at least three hours for digestion and should not take all the skins. Invariably, the best results have been effected when grapes have been taken in small amounts.

Some overzealous patients eat too many grapes. Two pounds a day, or if the patient is active and out of doors, three pounds, is usually enough. If the patient is not hungry, it is not necessary for him to force himself to eat. Seven meals a day is not compulsory nor is it necessary. Each case dictates its own conditions.

We have observed that the best results are obtained when the patients are given small quantities of grapes. Some patients are forced into eating too many grapes by anxious relatives. Sometimes one's loved ones are one's worst enemies at this stage of the diet. For that reason, it is well for the patient to go to a sanatorium,* if it is possible. Even though the patient

---

*[Sanatoriums, prevalent from 1840 to 1920, administered therapeutic treatments. Early sanatoriums were staffed by physicians and other medical specialists. Over time they evolved into retreats for relaxation, closer to our modern health spas. —C.V.]

should lose considerable weight, it does not mean that he is in danger of starving. The grape contains most of the food elements necessary to sustain life; many have been known to live many months on grapes, but this is not deemed advisable. Prudence and wisdom are essential; ill-timed zeal poses a serious threat to the patient.

A loathing for grapes may indicate the need for a fast—the presence of much poison in the system. Adding grapes or any other food to such a condition would, therefore, be injurious. The rule in such cases is to abstain from every form of food, drinking an abundance of cold water. Unless patients can eat the grapes with perfect enjoyment, they are better off without them. Skip a few meals. Let nature regulate this matter. *Loss of strength is due to the presence of poisons in the system.* The patient continues to weaken under the Grape Cure and under the complete fast until the poison has been expelled. Then, without a change of diet (and in case of a complete fast, without any food whatsoever), the patient often returns to strength and in some cases even puts on weight.

Ending the Regimen

If we could remove every trace of anxiety from the mind of the patient, the correct procedure would be to continue the exclusive grape diet until he stops losing weight. By watching the symptoms—the temperature, the excretions, eruptions, and so on—we know when the work of purification is complete. When this point has been reached—and it may last from two weeks to two months—it is advisable to go on to the second stage.

Reactions will be different in every case. It is therefore impossible to say beforehand how long it will be necessary to use grapes only. But this may be stated definitively—the cleansing of the alimentary canal takes time, and until this has been accomplished, the real relief does not begin. It is safe to say that the first seven to ten days on just grapes would be required to clear the stomach and bowels of their ancient accumulations. And it is during this period that distressing symptoms often appear. Nature works thoroughly. She does not build on a rotten foundation. The purification of every part of the body must be complete before new tissue can be built.

I think this is the only explanation of the excessive loss of weight under the Grape Cure. This question is of so much importance that we shall refer to it in detail concerning the treatment of cancer.

Meat is ruthlessly banned from this diet. Between meals, you can drink water or unsweetened herbal teas.

Possible Side Effects

FORMATION OF GAS

A development of which many complain in the Grape Cure is the formation of gas. When this symptom appears, it is good to stop the consumption of the skins altogether for a while. If this does not relieve the condition, one of the best remedies is a high colonic irrigation in the knee-chest position.*

SORENESS OF MOUTH

When the grape diet makes the mouth sore and raw, it may be because the flesh is diseased. Grapes do not have this effect on healthy tissue. When the body has been cleansed of its poisons, the soreness disappears.

---

*[Brandt is referring to a position in which the knees are brought up against the chest. Nowadays, colonic irrigation would be administered by a medical practitioner with modern, specialized equipment. —C.V.]

OTHER SYMPTOMS

Sometimes, after continuing on the grape diet for several weeks, the feces become quite black. This is also deemed a temporary symptom and no cause for any uneasiness.

Caution

Numerous instances have been reported of patients who have been misinformed as to the duration of the Grape Cure and the quantity of grapes to be consumed. This is regrettable because it detracts from the value of this wonderful discovery. The patient should be urged to adhere closely to the instructions given. The writer does not want to be held responsible for failures due to wrong advice by professional men who do not know anything about the Grape Cure.

The process of the grape when eaten exclusively tends to cleanse the intestinal tract and dissolve poisons that may have settled in any part of the body. Taking healing remedies is not recommended during the cure, unless they are homeopathic remedies.

THIRD STAGE: THE GRADUAL INTRODUCTION OF LIMITED FOODS

We do not expect anyone to live on grapes forever. The grape contains many of the most valuable elements necessary for life, but it does not contain everything. To live on grapes indefinitely would be to rob the system of some of the elements essential to life. When we are sure, therefore, that the grape has done its work by breaking up diseased tissue and purifying the blood, the careful introduction of other body-building foods is the next step. At the end of the exclusive diet, the stomach and digestive tube are still sensitive. Great care should be taken not to eat foods that are too rich.

Grapes should still form the main food and are always taken as the first meal in the morning and again at 8 PM. But now, during the day, some other fresh fruit may be used instead of grapes. An endless variety presents itself—a slice of melon, an orange, a grapefruit, an apple, a luscious pear, the scarlet strawberry, the golden apricot—one fruit more appetizing than the other.

Only one kind of fruit is to be taken at any meal, but something different every day.

After a few days, a glass of sour milk or buttermilk may be taken instead of grapes for dinner. Yogurt, fromage blanc, or cottage cheese can also be substituted for sour milk. Patients who dislike milk should take a ripe, firmly mashed banana or some other nourishing fruit.

After a week or ten days, every other meal may consist of different varieties of fruit or sour milk, taking them, for example, in the following order:

8 AM	Grape
10 AM	Pear, banana, or peach
12 PM	Grape
2 PM	Sour milk or buttermilk
4 PM	Grape
6 PM	Orange, grapefruit, plum, or apricot
8 PM	Grape

At this point, some patients crave something savory. The sweet fruits begin to pall. There may even be a positive aversion to grapes, in which case they should be omitted altogether and the other foods taken every three hours instead of every two.

One or two sliced tomatoes with pure olive oil and a little lemon juice may safely be included in this diet. The tomato is more of a berry than a vegetable, containing many valuable properties, and it forms an indispensable part of the diet in the third stage of the treatment.

FOURTH STAGE: THE RAW FOOD DIET

This includes every food that can be eaten uncooked—raw vegetables; salads; fruits; nuts; raisins, dates, figs, and other dried fruits; butter, cheese, cream, sour milk, and buttermilk; honey; and olive oil.

Begin the day as usual with cold water and grapes or some other fruit for breakfast, but instead of sour milk or fruit for lunch, have a substantial salad of raw vegetables. Reduce the number of meals, as raw vegetables take longer to digest.

It is surprising to some people to find that nearly all the vegetables can be used raw—young green peas and string beans, celery, tomatoes, cucumbers, lettuce, sprigs of cauliflower, squash, shredded cabbage leaves, grated carrots, turnips, beets and parsnips, finely chopped onions, and spinach.

After the light fruit diet, it is wise not to start out too soon with a large variety of vegetables. Choose two or three of the above-named as a foundation for your salad and mix them with lemon juice and olive oil. Try different varieties the following day and watch the combination of flavors.

Above all things, this noonday meal should be made palatable. Patients who have been used to animal food crave something stimulating. There can be no objection to adding one or two savory ingredients to this salad—some finely chopped nuts, grated cheese, sour cream, or a good mayonnaise made of eggs, lemon juice, and cold-pressed olive oil. Occasionally, a finely chopped hard-boiled egg can be added to the salad or served as an appetizer.

Time to Digest

Give this meal more time to digest than is required for raw fruits, especially if nuts, dates, raisins, or other dried fruits have been added to it.

The dinner should consist of sour milk, buttermilk, fromage blanc, or cottage cheese and fruits, or a highly nourishing and digestible dish may be made of mashed ripe bananas with sour cream.

Benefits of a Raw Food Diet

Raw foods contain an abundance of organic salts and vitamins. Sufficient stress cannot be laid upon the importance of the raw diet. If we could only educate the people about it, disease would be eradicated.

The raw foods digest more easily than the cooked and pass through the system far more rapidly. The result is that they have no time to decompose in the alimentary canal. There is no undue fermentation and no fear of poisoning.

I therefore strongly advise patients to abstain from every form of cooked food during the entire length of the treatment.

The course then consists of the four stages outlined above, and the highest results are obtained.*

But it is difficult, indeed, to convince people that they derive more nourishment from uncooked foods, and so we reluctantly consent to the introduction of one cooked meal a day. This is the fifth stage.

---

*[Whereas Brandt suggests that a raw food diet should be followed indefinitely, I recommend staying at the fourth stage for one week. —C.V.]

FIFTH STAGE: THE MIXED DIET

With this innovation, there is a recurrence of the old trouble in some cases, and the patient—sadder and wiser for the experience—is glad to go back to the raw diet. But if the disease has not been very deep-seated and the cure is complete, the following regimen is recommended.

Eat three meals a day:

1. A fruit breakfast, one kind only
2. A cooked lunch
3. A salad dinner

Single-Fruit Breakfast

For breakfast, eat plentifully of any of the juicy fruits that are in season. Make a strict habit of this and observe it for the rest of your life if you want to be healthy.

Skipping breakfast or having just a light breakfast of fruit is splendid for people who have been systematically overeating and especially those who are in the habit of indulging in heavy lunches and late dinners. But when the dinner is taken not later than 7 PM and consists of raw salad or fruit, the stomach of one who has been on a proper grape diet is free from acidity and accumulations.

In such cases, the fruit breakfast is better than the fast, in that it supplies the body with cleansing and building material.

One can, moreover, do a hard morning's work on a fruit breakfast.

The Cooked Meal

A dry meal. No soups (other than a good thick soup, which contains little liquid and is a meal in itself). No liquids of any kind.

No raw salads. No fruit either fresh or cooked.

The main foods are to be *steamed vegetables*. Begin with one kind at a time after the Grape Cure. If the results are good, take two or three varieties at a meal.

Not more than one kind of starch. This may consist of any of the cereals such as oatmeal and Wheatena, brown rice, potatoes, or whole wheat bread and unsalted butter.

Enjoy this meal. If you are not a vegetarian, indulge in a piece of baked, broiled, or steamed fish occasionally, with a steamed potato and butter. Or else, an infinite variety of savory dishes may be made by mashing one of the green vegetables with steamed potatoes, mixing it with egg, covering with bread crumbs and pats of butter, and baking this to a rich brown in the oven. Leftovers of cauliflower, cabbage, steamed lettuce, spinach, and baked onions lend themselves especially to this form of cooking. Take the time to arrange your dishes nicely, as visual pleasure is also important—the idea of sitting down to eat at the table should be inviting.

For variety, you can also prepare pasta or fresh corn on the cob or any of the other palatable food provided by nature.

Watch the effects of the cooked meal and with the first signs of discomfort, return to the raw diet.

CONCLUSION

To put it clearly, the condition of our blood is more dependent on the food we eat than on anything else, including thought. I know some saints whose bodies are very sick because they transgress against the laws of dietetics. And I know more than one sinner who is disgracefully healthy because he is more concerned about pure food than the good of his soul. Others there are, neither saints nor sinners, who have hardly had an original thought in their lives and yet are healthy and happy, like the cow placidly thinking of the next cud.

The thoughts of supermen may annul the effects of wrong eating, but until we reach that stage, we do well to study the daily menu.

When all is said and done, the matter of eating and drinking is at the present time the most important because it is the only thing over which we have conscious and deliberate control. We must concentrate on that, find out what are the best foods, and not allow ourselves to be persuaded by anyone to take anything that we know to be injurious.

A Summary of the Different Stages of Brandt's Grape Cure

First stage: The vital preparation before the cure—enemas and fasting

Second stage: The exclusive grape diet

Third stage: Gradual introduction of other raw fruits, tomatoes, sour milk, fromage blanc, cottage cheese, or yogurt

Fourth stage: The raw food diet

Fifth stage: The mixed regimen—a raw food diet with the introduction of some cooked foods

---

11

The Grape

THE MONO DIET

I believe it was the *exclusive grape* diet that saved my life in the end.

After the nine years' battle with death, I discovered almost accidentally that fresh grapes, *when taken alone,* answered the three requirements of dissolving, eliminating, and building.

Like everyone else, I had been eating grapes for years. I grew up among the vineyards of South Africa and the finest grapes of the world were to be found on our table at Harmony in Pretoria. We ate them with other foods. That was the mistake.

The stomach is nature's own laboratory. Put the right combination of foods into it and the result is the fabrication of every essence necessary for life and health.

But the stomach is also a still [apparatus used in distillation to produce alcohol]. At the temperature of blood heat, the process of digestion is carried on in the form of fermentation. The manufacture of alcohol can take place. This seems to be indispensable to the well-being of the body. But an excess of alcohol causes a poisoning of the system. Toxemia or autointoxication takes place. This is true when foods are mixed in the stomach indiscriminately, and especially so when to this mixture is added the grape. Taken into an impure stomach, it becomes a dangerous enemy.

On the other hand, when by fasting the system has been prepared for the change of diet, the grape becomes our great benefactor, our savior from the ills of the flesh.

The grape is, as far as I know, the most powerful nature solvent of chemical deposits, and at the same time the most drastic eliminator. Because of its extraordinary properties, the avenues of excretion become superbly active under a proper grape diet.

THE GRAPE AS FOOD AND MEDICINE

The medical properties of the grape cannot be overestimated. Salts of potash are found plentifully in grapes. And now we understand why the grape may be a specific cure for cancer, for there is said to be a marked deficiency of potash in the makeup of the average cancer patient.

The grape is remarkable. It is the finest natural tonic in the world. It also has some vital relation to the protein base of the protoplasm of the cell and is on that account considered a quick repairer of tissue waste. As a flesh- and muscle-forming element, it has no rival. In my opinion, the grape is a perfect food.

Proteins are the great body builders. This, then, partially explains why new tissue is built with such extraordinary rapidity on an exclusive grape diet.

But science has not yet discovered what elements in the grape break down malignant growths. Some fine essence, which has hitherto escaped observation, must be present in this "Queen of Fruits."

Perhaps this elusive substance will be found in the pure distilled water of the grape.

Supplemental Uses

We are only on the threshold of our discoveries and experiments, learning something new every day. With great success the pure juice of the grape is used for cleansing the throat, ears, nose, and mouth; applied externally on wounds in the forms of poultices and compresses diluted with water; and introduced per rectum as food. We can hope for yet more gifts from this queen of fruits.

GRAPE POULTICES

In the case of external growths, where there is an open sore, grape poultices have been found to be effective. The grape poultice is made by crushing grapes, spreading between layers of cheesecloth or muslin, and placing over the affected part, covering the whole with a dry cloth.

GRAPE COMPRESSES

Where whole grapes cannot be procured, a compress may be used. Soft muslin or cheesecloth is dipped in grape juice diluted about two-thirds. Both poultice and compress should be renewed frequently and the cloths safely disposed of, as they absorb much of the poison. The purpose of the compress is to keep external cancers and other wounds open and soft so that the poisons can be expelled. This is very important.

HEAD COLDS

Use also for sinusitis, brain fever, and similar ailments: a nasal douche six to eight times a day with diluted grape juice.

THROAT OR LARYNX CANCER
Gargle with diluted grape juice.

RECTAL CANCER
In addition to treating it with grapes as food, use diluted grape juice as an enema.

UTERINE CANCER
Regular injections of three parts lukewarm water and one part grape juice.

All the indicated treatments discussed in this section are to be performed as complements to the grapes ingested—in other words, as part of the Grape Cure. When the effects of the cure are too drastic (purgative), fast judiciously, then fast again—imbibing nothing but pure water. No lasting result can be obtained without fasting.

12

The Complements of the Grape Cure

THE DOCTORS OF NATURE

There are seven doctors of nature:

1. Fasting
2. Air
3. Water
4. Sun
5. Exercise
6. Food
7. Mind

Fasting

Fasting has already been discussed at length, so we will move right ahead to a description of the importance of air.

Air

Breathing well is essential because no one can renew the oxygen in one's lungs but oneself.

However, the respiratory tract is not the only thing

involved here: your skin is covered by millions of minuscule lungs: the pores. You must learn the magical effect of aeration and how to use an exfoliating body brush to stimulate the pores and rid them of accumulated inorganic substances.

The skin of a healthy person casts off the dead cells without artificial means, but in a diseased body the pores are choked with decayed matter. The entire body of the patient should be brushed morning and evening with a loofah or exfoliating brush.

These brushes may be procured at almost any drugstore or body care boutique.

But it is not enough to get the poisons out, you must see to it that no new poison gets in. There are more ways of taking in poison than through the mouth.

We do not put inorganic poisons into the system of a patient who is trying to expel poisons. That would be like pouring oil on a fire with one hand and water with the other, in an effort to extinguish it.

The construction of the human body is marvelously complex. The millions of pores on the surface have many functions. They not only excrete waste products, but they also have the power of absorbing material essences. The care of the skin is of immense importance in the treatment of cancer, for the pores are accessory organs of breathing. That is to say, instead of having only one pair of lungs, we possess many millions, so that in the case of internal cancer, when the breathing is heavily restricted, we have to depend largely on the free action of the pores for oxygen.

Individually, we have very little control over the air we breathe. But the human race is collectively responsible for the present tainted atmosphere by which the blood is poisoned. Until provision can be made to clear the air of smoke and gas and the deadly fumes of nicotine, our bodies will suffer. The annual cleansing by a thorough Grape Cure will be necessary.

Water

It would be impossible to fast for very long without using a lot of water, both internally and externally. Rainwater is surely the best choice. Distilled water can be used to drink for several weeks, but it is ill advised to make it a regular habit because it would deprive the body of certain mineral salts.

We have received many inquiries regarding the amount of water the patient should drink. The patient is permitted to drink as much water as he feels inclined to between the grape meals.

Generally, sufficient water is supplied by the juice of the grape. In the early stages of the diet, the patient often becomes very thirsty. Nature calls for an abundant supply of water to flush the system. After the poisons have been eliminated, this craving ceases. Too much drinking often tends to overwork the kidneys.

Ablutions, compresses, lotions, baths, body wraps, seawater baths, and ice cures all form part of this natural treatment. Make wide use of these methods by telling yourself that it is for your general well-being that you are devoting so much attention to your body.

Body wraps, water compresses, and poultices are highly commendable, and in extreme cases these should be saturated with diluted grape juice. A great many patients can now testify to the magical effects of these compresses.

Sun

Sunbathing can be combined with these methods. The vital emanations of the sun will be able to enter the body through the pores opened by the water. Caution: Don't expose yourself for too long or too quickly.*

Morning sunshine is the best. Don't lie out bare-headed. To be truly healthy, the sunbath should be taken gradually so that the skin pigmentation will darken normally. In order to take long sunbaths, you should wait until you have achieved a uniform tan.

Exercise

Life is movement. Death is stagnation. All forms of moderate exercise are good. We teach our students to gently massage the afflicted areas and to stretch their spinal column in order to improve the nervous system and blood circulation.

THE SACRED SPINE

Wonders have been accomplished with the Grape Cure, fasting, and the Fruitarian Diet, but the secret of perfect physical well-being lies in the condition of the spine. The bones should be well separated from one another by cushions of firm cartilage in order to allow an unrestricted flow of blood, nerve fluid, and other vital essences from the Generator of Life—the brain—to every part of the body.

The spinal column, or backbone, should be pliable, supple, and flexible without being limp; there should be no excessive curving in the lumbar region.

The full weight of the body should rest on the pelvis and be held in place by the internal muscles. This position tilts the pelvis forward and upward, lifts the ribs, expands the chest, reduces the abdomen, and lessens dangerous curves in the

---

*[Nowadays, because of our increased knowledge of the potentially harmful effects of the sun's rays and the hole in the ozone layer, extra caution should be taken. Protect yourself by wearing sunscreen. —C.V.]

lumbar region by the pressure of which the internal organs can be displaced, starved, and atrophied.

No living human being whose pelvic bones are out of place can breathe correctly or walk gracefully. Every movement becomes an effort. Wearing high heels is a prime culprit in the deformation of women's pelvises.

How can incorrect posture and the displacement of the pelvis be rectified?

There are many schools of physical culture teaching corrective exercises. There are trained chiropractors and osteopaths who, by the skillful manipulation of the spine, adjust the vertebrae and so release the pressure on the nerves.

Spinal extension and correction can also be obtained by suspension, based on the universal law of gravity.

All these exercises should be done under the supervision of a trained professional in a specialized institution.

We should remember, though, that in order to have perfect health, it is necessary to hold oneself properly and keep an eye on the state of one's spinal column.

Food

The healing that is possible with deliberate choices of the foods we take into our bodies has been sufficiently covered in other chapters.

Mind

It is the mind that cures. Man being a material being on a material plane, he requires material means to express his mind and spirit. The purification of the body acts directly on the mind, which, in turn, influences the habits of the body.

Mind operates through magnetism. In order, therefore, to contact the forces of mind, we purify and build up our personal magnetism. The best way to do this is to turn to the great doctors of nature.

THE PROMOTION OF HARMONY ON EARTH

The old method of reforming "the other fellow" is useless. We must begin with ourselves. We must start on the lowest vehicle—the physical body—and gradually work up to perfection of mind and spirit.

This is commonsense healing, or Harmony.

13

The Secret of the Success of the Grape Cure

SIMPLICITY

The Grape Cure is so simple that you can adopt it in your own home. It is only in extreme cases that patients are confined to their beds while on a grape diet. To be able to go about one's work as usual is perhaps one of the greatest advantages of this method. Think of what it means to the businesswoman, the professional man, the university student! Many have taken the exclusive grape diet and continued their work; sometimes it is advisable to take a short exclusive diet for the weekend and, after that, take the following three stages for an equal length of time, repeating this occasionally.

Power shall be added unto power. By the purification of blood and the general uplifting of mind and body resulting therefrom, I see the people of the earth gradually becoming more resistant to disease. Germs, plagues, and epidemics lose their terror. Fearlessness has been born. The entire mental outlook has been changed. Hopeful, constructive, optimistic, the sufferer sets about adjusting his faculties to this new psychology.

BLOOD DISEASES

There is said to be only one disease and that is blood disease. It is for the sake of convenience that we classify them into nervous, muscular, organic, or constitutional diseases. As a matter of fact—barring accidents and malformations—we depend, for life and health, largely on the condition of our blood. And our blood is dependent on what we think, on what we inhale, and on what we eat and drink.

PURIFYING THE BLOOD

I am convinced that cancer is a blood disease, more so, in fact, than any other disease. No bruise could develop into cancer if the blood was pure, and so I say again most earnestly, give the Grape Cure a trial! Go to the root of the matter and remove the cause of the trouble. Or better still, prevent future troubles.

There is nothing like the Grape Cure for purifying the blood from gouty and rheumatic poisons. The inorganic deposits that have settled between the joints are apparently dissolved and expelled in the form of diarrhea or as an unpleasant, oily sweat. The loosening of the joints sometimes causes great pain, which may be relieved by poultices or compresses of fresh grape juice.

THE COURSE OF THE DISEASE

Under the Grape Cure, cancer should run its full course within a month or six weeks. The patient loses weight to an extent that would be alarming if he did not understand the principle of the Cure. While on the first stages of the Grape Cure, nothing should be administered to make him gain weight—no food of any kind except the grape. In advanced cases of cancer, it is only by reducing him to a virtual skeleton that the disease may be overcome. When he has reached this point, when he has been brought almost to skin and bone, there is nothing left for the cancer to live on and it usually disappears spontaneously. There are many kinds of cancer, and the patients are all at different stages of the disease. It is therefore impossible to say beforehand how long it will take to arrive at the turning point.

NO CAUSE FOR ANXIETY

When the inorganic poisons have been effectively eliminated and the patient seems to have reached the last stage of weakness, there is usually a sudden and marked change for the better. He may fall into a refreshing sleep and wake up feeling "fine," feeling strangely invigorated—and usually his first demand is for "food." The greatest care must now be exercised. For a day or two, he should live on pure grape juice (homemade or unsweetened commercial)—half a pint sipped slowly every two hours, and then gradually the other fruits may be introduced.

The critical time is during that period of exhaustion just before the tide turns. It is so natural to think that the patient is dying for want of nourishment. This is not the case at all. If he has been kept faithfully on grapes, he has been fed with the finest and richest food on earth—a food that will sustain a healthy, active man for months.

"Feeding the patient to keep up his strength" is the surest way of killing him.

No, your cancer patient is not dying of starvation. And he is not getting weak because he is eating grapes only. But the cancer is dying. Nature is destroying it. The vital centers—heart, lungs, and brain—are being nourished to the last minute by the grape. To change the diet at this moment would compromise everything. Remember this when you are tempted to administer other foods and stimulants. His only chance may be the grape. You know the verdict that has been passed—inoperable cancer, no hope, nothing known to science that can save this case. Well, then, the grape is the only hope. Until you hear of something better than grapes, do not let the harrowing sight of the patient's weakness and emaciation tempt you to offer other foods. That might rob him of his only chance.

Give the grape diet a fair chance for a few weeks, not longer, if you are unable to get reliable advice. Then try some other juicy fruits.

I have seen patients reach the unconscious stage and then recover. Fortunately, the patients themselves often have a conviction that grapes and only grapes will save them.

To try them, I occasionally suggest some other tempting food and I have been impressed by the emphatic replies: "Not for a hundred thousand dollars!" or "I would rather die on grapes than live as I have been living on other foods."

The patients sense, before understanding, just what threatens their tortured bodies.

All this, however, applies only to the first few weeks of the exclusive grape diet. The danger of staying on grapes too long is that the patient may, in time, be unable to take any other food.

CURE DURATION

It has come to my attention that many patients overdo the exclusive grape diet. They seem to think they must continue the grape diet until the growth or other disorder has disappeared completely.

Experience teaches that scars caused by a malignant growth remain in the tissues long after the Grape Cure has done its work. Only time will show whether they will ever be entirely eradicated. The same is true of any injury done to the body through burns, cuts, fractures, etc. When the grape has purified the blood of cancer poison, the general condition of the patient steadily improves in spite of the presence of lumps, scars, or other evidence of the injury done by the growth.

In my own case, while the poisons of the cancer have been eliminated and the cancer has disappeared, physical examinations by medical men disclose that there are numerous adhesions as a result of the malignant growth. One doctor advances the opinion that it will take at least seven years for these adhesions to break up. It is useless, therefore, to continue the grape diet in the hope of completely eradicating the growth within a few weeks, or even a few months.

This treatment is slow, requiring patience and perseverance, but the patient is improving all the time, frequently able to go about his daily duties. One cannot expect to rid oneself within a few weeks of poisons that one has been *storing up one's entire life.*

Many patients who are employed and do not wish to become too greatly weakened take the exclusive grape diet for, say, two or three weeks; then they go on to the third and fourth stages for equal periods. If, at the end of that time, they feel that the poisons have not all been eliminated, they repeat the treatment. In that way, they are able to continue their employment.

The condition of each case should be watched carefully and judgment exercised. It is obviously impossible to give a set of rules that can be followed in each case.

The grape contains many of the elements necessary to

sustain life and health, but it does not contain everything. To continue the grape diet beyond a reasonable time would be to therefore deprive the system of the nourishment necessary for the maintenance of the body.

DO I NEED THE GRAPE DIET?

This is a question put most frequently. No one can answer it except yourself, and that is best done by starting right out on the diet. Try it for a week or two and at the end of that time you will probably know more about your condition than you ever did before.

The average person has been taught to regard every symptom of disease as an evil to be suppressed immediately. Nothing can be further from the truth. The disease is evil certainly, but the symptoms of disease are a curative process— not to be suppressed. This we find to be true under the fast and under every natural system of healing, but particularly so under the Grape Cure.

Abnormal growths, cancers, tumors, ulcers, abscesses, and fibrous masses seem to be dissolved by the powerful chemical agents in the grape. Diseased tissues and fatty degeneration, every form of morbid matter, is apparently broken up into minute particles and thrown into the bloodstream to be carried to the organs of excretion. No wonder, then, that complications arise. To the inexperienced person, it is disconcerting to find new symptoms of disease developing under the Grape Cure. He needs someone with experience to explain to him that poisons, which have been locked up in the system for many years, have broken loose and are running riot in the blood. Hence, that unusual rise of temperature, that eruption on the skin, those splitting headaches, those attacks of retching and purging, that discharge of mucus, that undue sweating.

The anxious mind of the patient should be set at rest by the assurance that all these are highly favorable symptoms of the process of purification being carried on internally—*proof positive that he is still vital enough to respond to the treatment.* The avenues of excretion—the bowels, kidneys, lungs, and skin—are still in good working order. Let him then closely examine the stools, the urine, the perspiration, and let him rejoice with the appearance of every new evidence that nature is still able to cast out the poisons that have been dislodged by the magical action of the grape. Pains and ailments are all a sign that nature is at work, purifying the body.

The patient should remember that every new ache and pain under the Grape Cure is an expression of life, of renewed activity. Nerves that have been atrophied for years have been stimulated by the grape.

Physical pain is Mother Nature's own voice warning us of danger. She speaks through the nerves, those delicate, watchful, and intelligent protectors of the human body.

So much depends upon his mental attitude that everything should be done to enlighten the patient on this most important aspect of the diet.

A volume could be dedicated to the remarkable effect of the grape upon the nervous system.

HEALING CRISES

No one can heal except nature. It is by the power of Mother Nature that we are healed. No one can renew the oxygen in one's lungs except oneself. Ignorance of these laws of nature keeps the world in the bondage of disease.

Your doctor may be puzzled by the strange actions and reactions—we call them healing crises—occurring under the Grape Cure. Then ask him to consult with someone who is experienced along these lines. The grape diet is very simple, but in cases of real danger, the first reactions may be highly complicated. Do not treat yourself without reliable advice.

A bad case of cancer of the tongue has been successfully treated, after a fast of ten days on water only, by the administration of a tablespoonful of grape juice every half hour.

Grape is the only nourishment prescribed in cases of enteric congestion. After a period of fasting, during which the system is cleaned and prepared for the change of diet, grape juice seems to act as a powerful disinfectant. At the same time, the strength of the patient is maintained by its nourishing properties.

Grapes apparently dissolve the hardened mucus adhering to the walls of the stomach and intestines. In several cases, along with the fecal matter, there was an accumulation of stringy, slimy mucus that resembled worms. Sometimes this occurred in long strings, sometimes in clumps resembling balls of string, and sometimes like black and green marbles. The grape juice appeared to dislodge this accumulation from the walls of the stomach and intestines and act as a flush, carrying it to the rectum. It is therefore considered very important to remove this accumulation by daily enemas, preferably high enemas (meaning those that penetrate deep into the colon). When taking only liquids, whether water or fruit juices, daily enemas are deemed necessary; otherwise, poisons that have been carried to the intestines by these liquids are likely to be reabsorbed into the blood.

KNOWING HOW
TO INTERPRET PROGRESS

The first results of the diet are different in every case. According to the condition of the patient, the first effects may be distressing or instantly beneficial. A healthy person may go on the exclusive grape diet and suffer no inconvenience, lose no weight, and be able to carry on his usual work without any loss of strength. Not so the sick. In a diseased body, the complications arising from the diet may be in exact accord with the gravity of the disease.

This is the perfect form of diagnosis and the most natural. It reminds me of the primitive test of the temperature of the baby's bath—when the baby turns red, the water is too hot; when the baby gets blue, the water is too cold. Poor baby! And one sometimes feels inclined to say "Poor patient!" when, under the Grape Cure, slumbering evils and latent diseases begin to manifest themselves. A seemingly healthy person may set out gaily on a grape diet—merely to reduce weight, for instance—and at the end of a few weeks, he may be quite a sorry spectacle. Some deep-seated trouble has been ferreted out into the open, and the wise thing to do in such a case is to continue the five stages of the diet until every trace of the disorder has disappeared.

OTHER DISEASES

It is impossible in a work of this scope to enumerate all the diseases that have been treated by this method. A few, about which special inquiries have come in, are mentioned below. I am also of the opinion that grapes should be the only food allowed to be consumed before and after an operation.

Arthritis

It stands to reason that when the bones have become ossified through arthritis and rheumatism, the Grape Cure will not loosen them up, except when used in conjunction with other methods of natural healing, such as manipulations, gentle exercise, and fomentation (the application of compresses). This should not be done without the supervision of one trained along these lines.

The patient should expect his pains to worsen, especially at the beginning of the cure. This is a normal reaction and proof that something constructive is happening.

Diabetes

This method has been particularly successful with diabetes. The grape sugar is believed to be an organic solvent that neutralizes the sugar deposits in the blood.

Patients used to taking insulin who devote themselves to the exclusive grape diet should reduce the dose of insulin until they are no longer taking any. One cannot expect satisfying results from the combination of insulin and grape juice.

[Caution: This should be done only under the supervision of the patient's doctor and with his or her consent.]

Gallstones

Gallstones have been cured while the patients were under treatment for more serious diseases.

Cataract

The same may be said of cataract of the eye.

Ulcerated Stomach

This must not be regarded lightly. Too often gastric ulcers, when neglected, become cancers. Before the disease reaches this point, it is highly recommended that the sufferer undergo the grape diet. In cases of this illness, the patient should not eat skins and seeds.

Pyorrhea Poisoning and Scurvy

The organic acids of the grape are strongly antiseptic and their effect on the gums is perhaps more valuable than any other result of the diet, for it means preservation of the teeth, on which mankind is dependent, not alone for health but for beauty as well.

Would that I had the tongue of a saint to warn against the evil of having sound teeth extracted because of poison at the roots! *It is not always necessary.* Every tooth may be loose in the socket and pus may be pouring from the gums, but after a few weeks on the exclusive grape diet, it will in time be found that the teeth are firmly set in the jaws and that every trace of pyorrhea poisoning has disappeared.

In my opinion, a patient suffering from scurvy should live exclusively on grapes for a certain length of time. *Try it. Prove it. Demonstrate the diet.*

Alcoholism and Addiction

The matchless grape is the supreme remedy for the craving of alcoholic liquors. Supplying, as it does, the purest form of the alcohol, which is indispensable to the maintenance of life and health, the grape should form the exclusive diet of our unfortunate fellow creatures addicted to drink as a preliminary measure before any other recovery methods are attempted.

And in our homes, every member of the family who is addicted to vice, to the drug habit, and to excessive use of tobacco, tea, and coffee would be persuaded to undergo a grape diet, without compulsion or threat. This hapless victim of perverted appetite is eager to be liberated. A sane and simple way of achieving this appeals to him.

INSTITUTIONS

What we need is an institution in which scientific work can be done along these lines, for the benefit of the world. To begin with, we need a well-equipped building in which cancer patients can be treated free of charge.

Does the amputation of a limb or the removal of an organ remove the cause of a cancer? Often a second operation becomes necessary. The cause of the trouble, I contend, is still in the blood.

The use of grapes can never restore the loss of limbs and organs, but painful swellings subside, inflammatory conditions are relieved, and there is an immense relaxation from nervous strain.

Again I plead for an opportunity to *demonstrate* these wonders.

Let the medical fraternity continue its research work. It is quite possible that it may some day hit upon something more effective than the grape diet.

APPEAL

Reader, are you going to do your share toward checking the devastating tide of disease and premature death that is spreading over the globe? Then do not be satisfied when, after the grape diet, you have regained perfect health. Your own freedom from suffering is not enough. Think of the other members of the human family and pass the message on. Tell your relatives and friends what the Grape Cure has done for you.

Final Thoughts on Brandt's Grape Cure

Ever since the time of antiquity, books have cited the healing properties of the grape, but none of these works emphasized the virtues of this fruit as out of the ordinary, nor did any propose grapes as a cure.

It was not until the second half of the nineteenth century—from 1840 to the First World War, to be precise—that what is now known as the Grape Cure experienced a boom in popularity. Health spas were created in the vineyard regions of Italy, Germany, and Switzerland, among other places. These healing centers—modeled on the thermal spa—welcomed cure seekers from all over Europe. Depending on the center and the era, the grape might compose the exclusive nourishment of people on the cure or it might appear as a complement to other therapies.

In the 1920s, in South Africa, a mother suffering from an incurable cancer desperately sought survival, a cure for her disease. Devouring every book on natural medicine she could find, experimenting on herself with all the healing procedures she had heard about from others, she eventually stumbled upon the healing properties of the grape, in the form of a mono diet. This mother was none other than Johanna Brandt.

Using the Grape Cure, she healed herself once and for all. After that, she took it upon herself to spread the word about the marvelous effects of this cure.

In her book, she placed the cure within everyone's reach, explaining how to follow the regimen. Little by little, her healing system spread; cure testimonies flooded in from all over, increasing the cure's renown.

The story of Brandt and the Grape Cure is typical of the empirical discovery of a healing procedure that becomes an accepted therapeutic system. The annals of natural medicine contain a host of similar examples. We should be grateful that new procedures of healing are constantly being discovered, adding to our therapeutic options. One cannot have enough strings for the bow when it comes to providing relief and healing! However, we should not lose sight of the fact that these procedures, even taken together, do not constitute natural medicine, properly speaking.

They may appear as such to those who are ill informed. In fact, these empirical procedures—whose efficacy requires no further demonstration, given the numerous testimonies of healing—are often considered universal healing techniques. As the testimonies demonstrate, procedures like these have effected cures for most known diseases, and many can be practiced as preventive measures, because they are seen as preventive, healing, and valid for themselves.

Yet, a medical system is not a collection of practical methods; it is an approach to health questions based on a *concept* of what illness is—a concept upon which practical procedures are developed. At the base of every medical system, there is a doctrine by which facts are interpreted and actions are oriented and directed.

Natural medicine, like all other therapies, has its own approach. The Grape Cure is not a doctrine, no more so than all the other procedures that have been discovered over the course of time. However, they are each practical illustrations of a piece of the doctrine. They demonstrate the soundness of the approach . . . each in its own aspect of the concept.

The ancient medical concept of health and disease—today called natural medicine—was formulated by Hippocrates. Despite periods when they fell into obscurity, the principles of this medical philosophy have survived into the present. The mind-dazzling progress of modern medicine might lead one to believe that, thanks to chemotherapy and the introduction of high technology into allopathic medicine, natural medicine has been struck a fatal blow. Nothing of the sort has happened. To the contrary, the abuses and excesses of the allopathic approach have only emphasized the necessity and importance of naturopathic medicine.

While every person in search of healing by natural means will profit by reading books like Brandt's, seekers must not stop there. They must also learn the basic principles of natural medicine to place such texts in their proper perspective in relation to the entire system of natural healing. Failing to do that, they will be walking blind, setting themselves up for failure, and possibly even destroying their health by misapplying techniques that are otherwise excellent in themselves.

The foundations of natural medicine as found in the writings of Hippocrates—who lived in the fourth century BCE—are presented in a manner difficult to understand in the modern world.

At the beginning of the twentieth century, however, Dr. Paul Carton reformulated the foundations of natural medicine, primarily in his *Traité de médecine, d'alimentation et d'hygiène naturiste* [Treatise on Naturopathic Medicine, Diet, and Hygiene], as well as in other works. With simplicity and logic—his books are written for the mass market—he explains the fundamental principles with all their implications for prevention and therapy, in domains as varied as diet, exercise, hydrotherapy, and more.

His expositions are so exhaustive they have become core works in the discipline. They continue to inspire and serve as references for medical practitioners the world over to such an extent that Dr. Carton can well be called the Hippocrates of the twentieth century.

By going beyond popular books on healing procedures and studying the foundations of natural medicine, you will discover it is more than a hodgepodge of herbal-tea recipes and miracle cures.

What you will find is a consistent and logical approach to health and disease, and thereby to humankind and life.

Notes

Foreword

1. Rosette Poletti, *Les soins infirmiers* [Nursing Care] (Paris: Le Centurion, 1978).

Chapter 1: The True Nature of Illnesses and Therapy

1. American Heart Association, http://www.americanheart.org/presenter.jhtml?identifier=4478, accessed April 24, 2006.

2. *Complete Works of Hippocrates,* French translation by Gardeil, Paris, volume 2, page 206.

3. Thomas Sydenham, *Practical Medicine* (n.p., n.d.).

4. Paul Carton, *Traité de médecine, d'alimentation et d'hygiène naturiste* [Treatise on Naturopathic Medicine, Diet, and Hygiene] (Paris: Éditions Maloine, 1924), 129.

5. *Complete Works of Hippocrates,* French translation by Gardeil, Paris, volume 1, page 143.

Chapter 2: Fasting

1. William D. Zoethout and W. W. Tuttle, *Textbook of Physiology* (St. Louis: The C. V. Mosby Company, 1946).

Chapter 5: The Raw Food Diet

1. Horace Fletcher, *The AB–Z of Our Own Nutrition* (New York: F. A. Stokes Company, 1903).

Chapter 6: Indications and Contraindications of the Grape Mono Diet

1. Paul Carton, *Traité de médecine, d'hygiène et d'alimentation naturiste* [Treatise on Naturopathic Medicine, Hygiene, and Diet] (Paris: Éditions Maloine, 1924).

2. *Complete Works of Hippocrates*, volume 2, page 32.

Resources

Author's Web Site
www.christophervasey.ch

The author presents his different books and provides for each of them the table of contents and a general introduction to the subject of the book. The Web site also contains biographical information, a calendar of events, and links to related sites.

SUPPLEMENTS

phion Nutrition
7741 E. Gray Road, Suite 9
Scottsdale, AZ 85260
888-744-8589
www.ph-ion.com

phion Nutrition is a manufacturer and distributor of products geared toward augmenting healthy body chemistry. Contact phion Nutrition or go to its Web site for further information about, or to order, the pH Test Strips mentioned in chapter 6.

Index

BOOKS OF RELATED INTEREST

The Acid-Alkaline Diet for Optimum Health
Restore Your Health by Creating Balance in Your Diet
by Christopher Vasey, N.D.

The Water Prescription
For Health, Vitality, and Rejuvenation
by Christopher Vasey, N.D.

The Whey Prescription
The Healing Miracle in Milk
by Christopher Vasey, N.D.

The Seasonal Detox Diet
Remedies from the Ancient Cookfire
by Carrie L'Esperance

The Tao of Detox
The Secrets of Yang-Sheng Dao
by Daniel Reid

The Clay Cure
Natural Healing from the Earth
by Ran Knishinsky

Food Combining for Health
Get Fit with Foods that Don't Fight
by Doris Grant and Jean Joice

Optimal Digestive Health: A Complete Guide
Edited by Trent W. Nichols, M.D., and
Nancy Faass, MSW, MPH

Inner Traditions • Bear & Company
P.O. Box 388
Rochester, VT 05767
1-800-246-8648
www.InnerTraditions.com

Or contact your local bookseller